Tuberculo

Arresting Everyone's Enemy

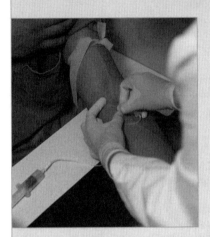

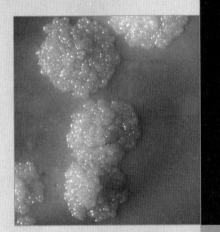

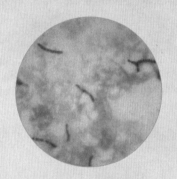

Joint Commission Resources

Second Edition

Senior Editor: Ilese J. Chatman
Project Manager: Andrew Bernotas
Manager, Publications: Paul Reis
Associate Director, Production: Johanna Harris
Associate Director, Editorial Development: Diane Bell
Executive Director: Catherine Chopp-Hinckley, Ph.D.
Vice President, Learning: Charles Macfarlane, F.A.C.H.E.
Joint Commission/Joint Commission Resources Reviewers: Patricia Adamski, Louise Kuhny, Linda Kusek, George Mills, Barbara Soule

Joint Commission Resources Mission

The mission of Joint Commission Resources is to continuously improve the safety and quality of care in the United States and in the international community through the provision of education and consultation services and international accreditation.

Joint Commission Resources educational programs and publications support, but are separate from, the accreditation activities of The Joint Commission. Attendees at Joint Commission Resources educational programs and purchasers of Joint Commission Resources publications receive no special consideration or treatment in, or confidential information about, the accreditation process.

The inclusion of an organization name, product, or service in a Joint Commission publication should not be construed as an endorsement of such organization, product, or service, nor is failure to include an organization name, product, or service to be construed as disapproval.

Printed in the U.S.A. 5 4 3 2 1

Requests for permission to make copies of any part of this work should be mailed to
Permissions Editor
Department of Publications
Joint Commission Resources
One Renaissance Boulevard
Oakbrook Terrace, Illinois 60181
permissions@jcrinc.com

ISBN: 978-1-59940-066-2
Library of Congress Control Number: 2007937066

For more information about Joint Commission Resources, please visit http://www.jcrinc.com.

Contents

Introduction

Tuberculosis is a common and deadly infectious disease caused by mycobacteria, mainly *Mycobacterium tuberculosis.* Tuberculosis most commonly attacks the lungs (as pulmonary tuberculosis), but can also affect the central nervous system, the lymphatic system, the circulatory system, the genitourinary system, bones, joints, and even the skin.

Although the tuberculosis rate in the United States declined in 2006 by 3.2% from the 2005 rate,[1] the disease is still a global threat, particularly in poverty-stricken populations. A reappearance of tuberculosis in the United States during the mid-1980s was successfully suppressed, but reappearance is always possible unless health care organizations, health care workers, government agencies, and the public maintain a high level of caution and awareness of the disease.

This book will help guide clinical leaders, laboratory directors, nursing home administrators, nurses, employee health leaders, staff educators, public health officials, risk managers, international infection prevention and control practitioners, and others involved in implementing tuberculosis guidelines in all types of health care settings. It also provides practical advice to help health care workers and hospitals, as well as other health care organizations, take a proactive and dynamic role in reducing the risk of a resurgence of tuberculosis in the United States.

Tuberculosis: A Historical Perspective

Tuberculosis has been with us since prehistoric times. Distinguishing lesions in prehistoric skeletons and Egyptian mummies reveal the disease. The spinal form of tuberculosis (also known as Potts disease) was particularly prevalent in ancient Egypt.

Written descriptions of tuberculosis symptoms—bloody cough, night sweats, fevers, and appetite and weight loss—can be found in ancient writings. The

As Europe emerged from the Dark Ages, a renewed interest in science and art coincided with an epidemic of tuberculosis that began in early 1600 and continued for the next two centuries. Increased population centers, accompanied by poverty, contributed to this epidemic. Tuberculosis became known as the White Death, and was almost as feared as the Black Death, also known as bubonic plague.

ancient Greeks were scientifically intelligent and wrote about many diseases, including tuberculosis. In fact, Hippocrates is credited with first using the term *phthisis* (meaning wasting or consumption) for the disease, which for hundreds of years was the most common term used.

During the eighteenth, nineteenth, and early twentieth centuries, tuberculosis was romanticized. The disease was called *consumption* because of the appearance of the body being consumed from within. It became almost glamorous to look frail and sickly, and the disease was thought to affect artistic and romantic personalities. This seemed to be validated by the fact that many creative people in literature and the arts during that time were afflicted with the disease. The poet John Keats, also a physician, realized his illness when he began coughing up blood at the age of 23. During the previous year Keats nursed his younger brother Tom through the terminal stages of the disease, which had ended Tom's life only a few months before Keats became ill. Keats lived three more years, and was as much afflicted by the treatment as the disease itself. Keats tried bloodletting, starvation, antimony (a harmful toxic metal), and a prescription of horseback riding, which were all treatments tried by physicians of that time.

Other artists also died of consumption during this period, including French playwright Moliere; Italian composer Giovanni Battista Pergoleso; English writer Laurence Sterne; poet Percy Bysshe Shelley; painters Tom Girtin, Joseph Mallard William Turner, and Richard Parkes Bonnington; composer Frederic Chopin; and many others. The disease took a particularly hard toll on the Bronte family: All of the siblings died of the disease, including authors Branwell, Emily, Anne, and Charlotte. During this time, persons with consumption were the subjects of plays, operas, paintings, and novels, including a novel by Alexandre Dumas *fils* that later became the opera *La Traviata* and the Greta Garbo film *Camille*.[2]

The reality of tuberculosis, however, is far less glamorous. At the time, it was primarily a disease of poverty, which is often accompanied by overcrowding, inadequate ventilation, and malnutrition. There was also a higher infectivity rate for persons who nursed and cared for consumption patients. Tuberculosis became a significant killer of the poor and young in England during the early 1800s. This coincided with the Industrial Revolution, and the decline of the disease since 1840 is considered to be a return to the pre–Industrial Revolution level. A major contributing factor to the spread of the disease occurred around the year 1800, when children began to be commonly exploited for labor in factories.

From the middle of the nineteenth century, we have data of sorts for Britain, Ireland, continental Europe, and North America. Interesting aspects of the data include the following:

- Significant differences were found to exist between adjacent impoverished and more affluent neighborhoods in London. At least half the infant deaths in poor neighborhoods were credited to phthisis or lung disease.
- In Dublin, which was very impoverished, the mortality rate from phthisis in the 1880s was almost twice as high as the overall mortality rate in London.
- Of the autopsies performed on children dying of all causes in the London Hospital for Sick Children in the 1880s, tuberculosis was recorded as the principle cause of death in approximately 45% of those cases.
- Every winter between 1870 and 1890 half of all prisoners in Chatham Naval Prison developed tuberculosis and died.
- After prisons, the next highest incidence of endemic tuberculosis was in the houses of European female religious orders. As one example, nearly two thirds of the deaths in 38 Prussian nursing convents between 1864 and 1889 were attributed to tuberculosis.

Although physicians throughout these times were attempting to find the source of the disease and curative treatments, they were still essentially following the advice of the ancient Greek physician Galen, who had prescribed "fresh milk, open air, sea breezes, and dry mountainous places." In the nineteenth and twentieth centuries, sanatoriums were established for those who could afford them to allow recuperative rest in a healthier climate.

In the mid-1800s many researchers experimented with finding the source of various diseases, including tuberculosis. In 1881, Robert Koch, who was the first to culture the anthrax bacillus, began his work on tuberculosis. Koch used a four-step method to prove that bacteria caused the disease. The tuberculosis bacteria were isolated from animals that had the disease; the bacteria then were grown through culturing. Next, Koch injected the cultured organisms into healthy animals, which later became ill and died. Koch then recovered and identified tuberculosis bacteria from those animals. The word *tuberculosis* was later labeled as the ailment because of the appearance of tubercles (tumor-like nodules) that appear as the tuberculosis bacteria multiply in clusters.

When Koch announced his findings, it shocked the scientific community because many assumed that consumption was an inherited disease. Thirteen years later, William Roentgen discovered x-rays. With the x-ray machine, clinicians were able to have a picture of the scar tissue and inflammation caused by tuberculosis.

Although tuberculosis was more common among immigrants and the poor, public health officials realized that everyone was vulnerable due to the fact that it is spread through the air. Therefore, they began campaigns to reduce the spread of the disease.

In 1893 Dr. Hermann Biggs in New York City published a report recommending an education campaign, the separation of tuberculosis patients in hospitals, the establishment of a special hospital for tuberculosis patients, the disinfection of homes or hospital rooms of tuberculosis patients, and the diagnostic examination of sputum in

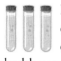 In 1887 Sir Robert W. Phillip put into place the first tuberculosis control program in Edinburgh, Scotland. Sir Phillip's system encompassed many of the processes used today in good public health programs, including the following:

- Aggressive diagnosis
- Required reporting of tuberculosis patients to public health authorities
- Record keeping
- Testing (examination of sputum for tuberculosis bacteria)
- Public education
- Social services
- Home visits by doctors and nurses
- A dispensary
- Follow-up care

patients with pulmonary disease. Biggs also promoted a requirement for clinicians to report all tuberculosis cases to the health department. Today, tuberculosis is still reportable to public health authorities to protect the public.

By the beginning of the twentieth century, doctors could diagnose tuberculosis disease easily, but there was no way to cure it. Although various vaccines were tried, they were less than satisfactory, and it wasn't until antibiotics became available that the treatment for tuberculosis would change. In 1943 Selman Waksman discovered streptomycin. In 1944 streptomycin was used at the Mayo Clinic on a tuberculosis patient who was near death. The patient received many injections of streptomycin, with later injections being of higher concentration. The patient recovered and lived a normal life. However, for other patients, the results were mixed. Many would seem to recover, but would then relapse. There were some people who were able to live with the disease in an inactive stage as a result of using streptomycin.

Para-aminosalicylic acid became available for clinical use in 1946, isoniazid in 1952, pyrazinamide in 1961, ethambutol in 1963, and rifampin in 1966. These antibiotics proved to be very effective against the disease, and patients who had previously been given a 50% chance of survival would feel better in a matter of weeks after treatment. The solution: Patients needed to keep taking the medication much longer after they felt well, or they would often have a relapse. These antibiotics proclaimed a new era in the fight against tuberculosis.[3]

Tuberculosis Today

Today, tuberculosis continues to present new public health challenges, particularly with the advent of drug-resistant strains of the disease, as well as increased vulnerability to tuberculosis for those with immune system deficiencies such as human immunodeficiency virus (HIV). In addition, experts warn that as the incidence of tuberculosis declines in the United States, fast and accurate diagnosis of symptoms may also wane. In an effort to reduce complacency, the Centers for Disease Control and Prevention (CDC) now recommend that the fight against tuberculosis be expanded to include settings outside of the traditional hospital milieu.

The World Health Organization's (WHO) Stop TB Partnership's *The Global Plan for 2006–2015* recommends that strategic actions be implemented to combat tuberculosis worldwide. The global plan embraces the WHO concept of controlling this disease by using the following summarized action activities:

1. Practice superior *directly observed therapy, short course* (DOTS) to improve the ability to diagnose tuberculosis cases and to help identify cures through a patient safety–centered focus and approach that reaches all patients, particularly the poor.
2. Concentrate on tuberculosis/HIV, multidrug-resistant tuberculosis and other problems by ramping up tuberculosis/HIV combined-care actions, DOTS, and other relevant patient-focused activities.
3. Contribute to strengthening health care systems by collaborating with other health care programs and organizations.
4. Involve all health care providers, the public, nongovernmental agencies, and private organizations by ramping up methods to guarantee observance of international standards associated with patient care of tuberculosis.
5. Involve people with tuberculosis and people living in communities that are affected by tuberculosis by promoting medical contributions to effective care. This could entail ramping up communitywide tuberculosis care and services, communicating various topics associated with the disease, and supporting an agreement between patients and their communities.
6. Allow and encourage research for the development of new drugs, diagnostics, and vaccines.

More information on WHO's "The Global Plan to Stop TB" can be found in Chapter 5, pages 129–134.

Directly Observed Therapy (DOT)

Directly observed therapy (DOT) is an adherence-enhancing strategy in which a health care worker or trained person watches a patient swallow each dose of medication. DOT is the standard care for all patients with tuberculosis disease and is a preferred option for patients with treated latent tuberculosis infection.

Directly Observed Therapy, Short Course (DOTS)

Directly observed therapy, short course (DOTS) is a comprehensive adherence-enhancing strategy that includes DOT as well as additional methods to promote treatment adherence, such as providing support and care that emphasizes the needs of the individual patients and their families and finding locally appropriate ways to motivate patients to participate in and complete their tuberculosis treatment.

Content of This Book

Tuberculosis: Arresting Everyone's Enemy, Second Edition, explains the latest edition of the CDC's "Guidelines for Preventing the Transmission of *Mycobacterium tuberculosis* in Health-Care Facilities, 2005," and what health care organizations can do to implement the new recommendations, with an expanded focus on various health care settings.

Chapter 1: What Health Care Workers Need to Know About Tuberculosis

Chapter 1 provides an overview of tuberculosis and its various forms, the potential for tuberculosis transmission, and populations that are paticularly at risk. It also summarizes the CDC guidelines and the expanded focus on health care settings such as hospitals; long term care, ambulatory care, and home care settings; emergency medical services; physicians' and dentists' offices; clinical laboratories; behavioral health care programs; and correctional facilities.

Chapter 2: Early Identification and Isolation of Infectious Individuals

Chapter 2 reviews current strategies and protocols for diagnosis, isolation, and treatment of tuberculosis. It also describes the protocols for conducting tests in populations that continue to have tuberculosis infection rates that are greater than the U.S. average.

Chapter 3: Infection Control

Chapter 3 includes detailed information on administrative, environmental, and respiratory protection controls that health care facilities must use to prevent the spread of tuberculosis infection among patients, visitors, and health care workers. This includes steps for conducting risk assessments in your organization to determine the levels of controls required and for addressing infection incidents as they occur.

Chapter 4: Patient, Visitor, and Health Care Worker Education

Chapter 4 provides tools and strategies for educating patients regarding infection and treatment, educating family members and visitors regarding risks, following respiratory precautions, and educating staff to identify symptoms.

Chapter 5: International Implications

Chapter 5 discusses tuberculosis trends worldwide, along with the WHO's "Stop Tuberculosis Strategy." Worldwide trends are important because the increase in immigration from countries where tuberculosis is more prevalent is a significant concern in the United States' fight against tuberculosis.

Various definitions can be found throughout the book 🐷 as well as in the Glossary. An Index is also provided.

Acknowledgements

Joint Commission Resources would like to thank Marilyn Sims and Julie Chyna for their indispensable writing skills and contributions to the content of this book. We also thank Joint Commission reviewers Patricia Adamski, Louise Kuhny, Linda Kusek, and George Mills, and Joint Commission Resources' Infection Control Practice Leader, Barbara Soule, for their indispensable knowledge and insight on this topic.

References

1. Centers for Disease Control and Prevention: Trends in tuberculosis incidence—United States, 2006. *MMWR Morb Mortal Wkly Rep* 56:245–250, Mar. 23, 2007.
2. Dormandy T.: *The White Death: A History of Tuberculosis.* New York: New York University Press, 2000, pp. 13–22, 76–81.
3. Reichman L.B., Tanne J.H.: *Timebomb: The Global Epidemic of Multi-Drug-Resistant Tuberculosis.* New York: McGraw-Hill, 2002, pp. 23–39.

Chapter 1

What Health Care Workers Need to Know About Tuberculosis

What Is Tuberculosis?

The American Lung Association defines tuberculosis as an airborne infection caused by the bacterium *Mycobacterium tuberculosis* that primarily affects the lungs. Tuberculosis can be spread by coughing, sneezing, laughing, or singing. Repeated exposure to someone with tuberculosis disease is generally necessary for infection to take place. Although tuberculosis primarily affects the lungs, other organs and tissues may be affected as well. Sidebar 1-1, page 11, provides more detail on other mycobacterial species. Although tuberculosis can be readily treated and prevented, it continues to be a very serious public health problem in many areas of the world.

A majority of persons infected with *M. tuberculosis* do not become physically ill with the disease, but rather have a condition known as latent tuberculosis infection (LTBI). A person with LTBI does not have the tuberculosis disease, but some of the bacteria can remain viable for years. The person's immune system keeps the infection in this inactive state, but when the immune system becomes challenged in any way, the possibility for an escalation to the disease state increases dramatically.

Elimination Plan

In 1989 the Centers for Disease Control and Prevention (CDC) published *A Strategic Plan for the Elimination of Tuberculosis in the United States*. This plan proposed a strategy for eliminating tuberculosis by 2010, but a resurgence of the disease in the late 1980s and early 1990s hindered the plan's fulfillment. The resurgence was attributed to a combination of factors, including the onset of the human immunodeficiency virus/acquired immunodeficiency syndrome (HIV/AIDS) epidemic, increases in tuberculosis cases among non–U.S.-born persons, tuberculosis outbreaks in congregate settings, and the appearance and transmission of deadly multidrug-resistant tuberculosis (MDR-TB) strains.[1] Because of these complications, the CDC commissioned the National Academy of Sciences' Institute of Medicine to determine if tuberculosis elimination in the United States is still feasible. The study concluded that tuberculosis elimination is feasible, but will require decisive and aggressive action beyond what is now in effect.

As a response, the CDC published the "Guidelines for Preventing the Transmission of *Mycobacterium tuberculosis* in Health-Care Facilities, 1994." The implementation of these guidelines in health care facilities in the United States produced the desired effect—a decrease in the number of tuberculosis outbreaks in health care settings and a reduction in health care–associated transmission of *M. tuberculosis* to patients and health care workers. At the same time, the nation's tuberculosis control programs succeeded in reversing the upsurge of tuberculosis cases, and case rates continued to decline over the subsequent 10 years. The threat of MDR-TB is decreasing, and transmission of *M. tuberculosis* in health care settings continues to decrease. However, recorded declines in tuberculosis rates in the United States in 2003 and 2004 were the lowest recorded since 1993. In addition, tuberculosis infection rates greater than the U.S. average continue to be reported in certain racial/ethnic populations. Therefore, the CDC reevaluated and updated the guidelines for health care settings in 2005 in order to define actions to continue the momentum attained since 1994. These "Guidelines for Preventing the Transmission of *Mycobacterium tuberculosis* in Health-Care Settings, 2005," were published in the December 30, 2005, issue of *Morbidity and Mortality Weekly Report.* The CDC continues to update this and other information as necessary.

At the same time, the World Health Organization (WHO) developed *The Global Plan to Stop TB 2006–2015* in close collaboration with partners worldwide. This campaign aims to dramatically reduce the global burden of tuberculosis by 2015 by

In a report published on March 24, 2006, *Morbidity and Mortality Weekly Report* noted that the CDC, in collaboration with the WHO and participating supranational reference laboratories, had agreed to define extensively drug-resistant tuberculosis (XDR-TB) as cases of tuberculosis disease in persons whose *M. tuberculosis* isolates were resistant to both isoniazid and rifampin and to at least three of the six main classes of second-line drugs (aminoglycosides, polypeptides, fluoroquinolones, thioamides, cycloserine, and para-aminosalicyclic acid).

Health Care Workers
All paid and unpaid persons working in health care settings.

improving access to high-quality diagnosis and treatment and enabling and promoting research.[2] (For more information on this campaign, *see* Chapter 5.)

Both strategies recognize that the risk factors for tuberculosis are very complex and include socioeconomic factors as well as infection control issues.

Tuberculosis Trends in Recent Years

Since 1953 the CDC has collected information on the number of newly reported tuberculosis cases in the United States. The data since then have shown a steady decline in the number of tuberculosis cases reported, as well as in deaths due to tuberculosis, until the mid-1980s, when the numbers began to climb. Factors contributing to this increase include the following[3]:

- Deterioration of the tuberculosis public health infrastructure during that time
- The HIV/AIDS epidemic
- Increase in numbers of people immigrating from countries where tuberculosis is common
- Transmission of tuberculosis in congregate settings, such as correctional facilities, homeless shelters, and health care facilities

Sidebar 1-1.
Other Species of Mycobacteria

Three other closely related mycobacterial species can cause tuberculosis disease, and along with *M. tuberculosis,* make up the *M. tuberculosis* complex. These are *M. bovis, M. africanum,* and *M. microti. M. microti* does not cause disease in humans; the other two mycobacteria are found very rarely in the United States. Mycobacteria other than these that make up the *M. tuberculosis* complex are called nontuberculous mycobacteria, and may cause pulmonary disease resembling tuberculosis.

In 1989 the CDC announced a goal to eliminate tuberculosis from the United States by 2010 and published the *Strategic Goal for the Elimination of Tuberculosis in the*

United States. The goal and document were reassessed in 1999 to identify actions required to achieve the original goal. This attention on tuberculosis, along with another task force that convened in 1992 on combating MDR-TB and the publication of the "Guidelines for Preventing the Transmission of *Mycobacterium tuberculosis* in Health-Care Facilities, 1994," focused public health and other medical professionals on the need to increase clinical knowledge about tuberculosis infection and the disease. This has resulted in more expeditious identification of persons with tuberculosis, a greater rate of appropriate treatment, and increased efforts to ensure that patients complete the therapy.

Since 1993 tuberculosis case rates for U.S.-born and non–U.S.-born persons have been declining, which indicates that reduction efforts have helped to reverse the upward trend of tuberculosis that occurred in the mid-1980s. Figure 1-1 (page 13) and Table 1-1 (page 14) show the downward trend since 1993.

In the United States, reports of tuberculosis cases are made to the CDC by each of the 50 states, the District of Columbia, New York City, Puerto Rico, and seven other jurisdictions in the Pacific and Caribbean. Figure 1-2, page 15, shows the breakdown of tuberculosis cases by state, and Figure 1-3, page 16, shows the breakdown by race/ethnicity.

A summary of the data analysis for 2006 includes the following[4]:
- A total of 13,767 cases were reported, a 3.2% decrease from 2005.
- California, Florida, Georgia, Illinois, New Jersey, New York, and Texas account for 60% of the 2006 national tuberculosis case total.
- Among persons with tuberculosis whose country of birth was known, 74.7% of Hispanics and 29.9% of non-Hispanic blacks were foreign born.
- Asians and Native Hawaiians or other Pacific Islanders continue to have the highest case rate (number of cases per 100,000 population) among all ethnic/racial groups.
- Nineteen states, including the District of Columbia,. reported an increase in rates.
- The top five countries of origin of non–U.S.-born persons with tuberculosis were Mexico, the Philippines, Vietnam, India, and China.

Other information determined from the data analysis includes statistics on the number of XDR-TB cases under the revised definition:
- Since 2000, the proportion of patients with primary MDR-TB has remained the same at 2.0%.

Figure 1-1. Reported Tuberculosis Cases in the United States, 1993–2006

The resurgence of tuberculosis in the mid-1980s was marked by several years of increasing case counts until it peaked in 1992. Case counts began decreasing again in 1993, and 2006 marked the 14th year of decline in the total number of tuberculosis cases reported in the United States since the peak of the resurgence. From 1992 until 2002, the total number of tuberculosis cases decreased 5% to 7% annually. From 2002 to 2003, however, the total number of tuberculosis cases decreased by only 1.4%. In 2006 a total of 13,767 cases were reported from the 50 states and the District of Columbia. This represents a decline of 3.2% from 2005.

Number and Rate (per 100,000) of Tuberculosis Cases—U.S.-Born and Non–U.S.-Born Persons—United States 1993–2006*

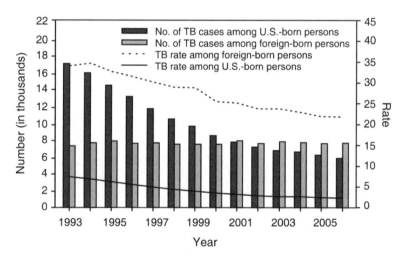

* Data for 2006 are provisional.

Source: Centers for Disease Control and Prevention: Trends in tuberculosis incidence—United States, 2006. *MMWR Morb Mortal Wkly Rep* 56, Mar. 23, 2007. http://www.cdc.gov/mmwR/preview/mmwrhtml/mm5611a2.htm (accessed Sep. 12, 2007).

Table 1-1. Tuberculosis Morbidity: United States, 2000–2006

Year	Cases	Rate per 100,000 Population
2000	16,309	5.8
2001	15,946	5.6
2002	15,056	5.2
2003	14,840	5.1
2004	14,515	4.9
2005	14,085	4.8
2006	**13,767**	**4.6**

Source: Centers for Disease Control and Prevention: Trends in tuberculosis incidence—United States, 2006. *MMWR Morb Mortal Wkly Rep* 56, Mar. 23, 2007. http://www.cdc.gov/mmwr/PDF/wk/mm5611.pdf (accessed Sep. 12, 2007).

- During the years 2000–2006, the proportion of U.S.-born patients with MDR-TB has decreased from 59% in 1993–1999 to 24%. However, the percentage of non–U.S.-born patients with MDR-TB has increased from 38% in 1993–1999 to 76% from 2000–2006.

Although the data show an overall decrease in tuberculosis cases, there is concern about the fact that the proportion of tuberculosis cases among non–U.S.-born persons has increased steadily since the mid-1980s and has increased markedly since 1992.

What These Trends Mean for Caregivers and Organizations

The overall decrease in tuberculosis cases and MDR-TB that has occurred since 1992 is definitely encouraging. However, the health care profession cannot afford to grow complacent: A false sense of security was partly to blame for the 1980s resurgence. All health care departments and organizations need to be prepared for prompt identification of active tuberculosis disease and implementation of isolation and treatment.

Information from this statistical data can be used along with guidelines and evidence-based practices in developing programs for each health care setting's tuberculosis risk and in maintaining the ability to readily identify and treat people who are infected with *M. tuberculosis.* The last section of this chapter gives practical advice for meeting guidelines in various health care settings.

Figure 1-2. Tuberculosis Case Rates per 100,000 Population, United States, 2006

This map shows the rate of tuberculosis (TB) cases for the 50 U.S. states and the District of Columbia (DC). In 2006, for the second consecutive year and the second time since national reporting began, approximately half of states (26 of 50) had TB rates of < 3.5 per 100,000 persons; however, 11 of those 26 states had higher rates of TB in 2006 than in 2005.

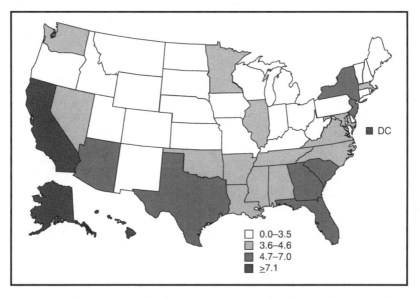

Source: Centers for Disease Control and Prevention: Trends in tuberculosis incidence—United States, 2006. *MMWR Morb Mortal Wkly Rep* 56, Mar. 23, 2007. http://www.cdc.gov/mmwr/PDF/wk/mm5611.pdf (accessed Sep. 12, 2007).

Disease Transmission

Tuberculosis is spread through the air. For transmission to occur, a person with pulmonary or laryngeal tuberculosis must cough, sneeze, speak, or sing, and in doing so, expel and disperse droplet nuclei containing *M. tuberculosis* into the air. Normal air currents can keep these particles airborne for prolonged time periods and spread them throughout a room or building. Depending on the environment, these tiny particles can remain suspended in the air for several hours. The bacteria are usually transmitted only through air and not by surface contact.[5]

Figure 1-3. Tuberculosis Case Rates* by Race/Ethnicity[†]— United States, 2005–2006[‡]

Asians, American Indian/Alaska Natives, and Native Hawaiian and Pacific Islanders show a decline in tuberculosis rates between 2005 and 2006 (22.6%). Among non-Hispanic blacks or African Americans, rates declined from 10.9% in 2005 to 10.1% in 2006; among Hispanics, from 9.5% to 9.2%; and among non-Hispanic whites, from 1.3% to 1.2%.

Race/Ethnicity	2005		2006		% change 2005–2006		Population	
	No.	Rate	No.	Rate	No.	Rate	2005	2006
Hispanic	4,047	9.5	4,050	9.2	0.1%	-3.0%	42,687,224	44,046,771
Black	3,955	10.9	3,712	10.1	-6.1%	-7.1%	36,324,593	36,693,014
Asian	3,209	25.8	3,269	25.6	1.9%	-1.0%	12,420,514	12,779,154
White	2,579	1.3	2,404	1.2	-6.8%	-7.0%	198,366,437	198,819,462
American Indian/Alaska Native	152	6.8	164	7.3	7.9%	6.6%	2,232,922	2,259,052
Native Hawaiian or Other Pacific Islander	53	13.1	62	15.1	17.0%	15.0%	405,019	411,932
Multiple race	46	1.2	38	0.9	-17.4%	-19.8%	3,973,695	4,093,276
Unknown	44	—	68	—	—	—	—	—
Total[¶]	14,085	4.8	13,767	4.6	-2.3%	-3.2%	—	—

* Per 100,000 population.

[†] Persons identified as White, Black, Asian, and of other or unknown races are all non-Hispanic. Persons identified as Hispanic might be of any race.

[‡] Data for 2006 is provisional.

[¶] Total rates were calculated by dividing the total number of reported cases by the total U.S. Census population, then multiplying by 100,000.

Source: Centers for Disease Control and Prevention: Trends in tuberculosis incidence—United States, 2006. *MMWR Morb Mortal Wkly Rep* 56, Mar. 23, 2007. http://www.cdc.gov/mmwr/PDF/wk/mm5611.pdf (accessed Sep. 12, 2007).

Not everyone who inhales the bacteria becomes infected, and in fact, there is only a 25% chance of infection. However, a susceptible person may become infected when droplet nuclei containing *M. tuberculosis* are inhaled and pass through the mouth or nasal passages, upper respiratory tract, and bronchi to reach the alveoli. Most of the larger particles become lodged in the upper respiratory tract, where infection is less apt to develop; however, the smaller particles have a greater chance of reaching the alveoli, where infection can take hold.

After the particles are in the alveoli, the tubercle bacilli are ingested by macrophages; most of the bacteria are destroyed or inhibited. However, a small number are able to multiply within the macrophages and then are released when the macrophages die. In some cases, local infection may occur, followed by dissemination to the lymphatic and circulatory systems, which can spread the infection throughout the body.

In most cases, within 2 to 12 weeks of the initial infection, the person's immune response will limit multiplication of the bacilli, but will not destroy all of them. Some will remain in the body and be viable for many years. When this occurs, the person has LTBI. People with LTBI have no symptoms of and are not considered to have tuberculosis. In addition, those with LTBI are not infectious and cannot transmit the disease unless they develop symptoms.

Unless persons with LTBI are treated, a certain percentage will develop tuberculosis disease. In the United States, approximately 5% of untreated persons with LTBI will develop the disease within the first two years after infection has occurred. Another 5% of untreated infected people will develop the disease sometime in their lives. There are some medical conditions that increase the risk that LTBI will progress to disease. One such disease is HIV, which is the strongest known risk factor for development of tuberculosis disease in people who have LTBI.

Tuberculosis is most commonly found as a pulmonary infection: 73% of tuberculosis cases are exclusively pulmonary. Persons with this type of tuberculosis are likely to be infectious.

However, tuberculosis is a systematic disease and may also occur in the following areas:
• The bones and joints
• The central nervous system
• The lymphatic system
• The genitourinary system
• As a pleural effusion
• More rarely in other body sites, such as the breast, skin, or peritoneum

Extrapulmonary tuberculosis is more common in persons who are immunosuppressed and in young children. It is also often associated with pulmonary tuberculosis. The term *miliary tuberculosis* refers to a rarely occurring combination of extrapulmonary and pulmonary tuberculosis.

Infectivity Risks and Epidemiology

Those at higher risk of exposure to or infection with *M. tuberculosis* are close contacts of someone who has active pulmonary tuberculosis disease. These are people who share the same household or other enclosed spaces. Because such people are usually family members, the disease was once thought to be genetic.

Others at high risk of exposure include the following[6]:
- Non–U.S.-born persons (including children) from areas where tuberculosis is common, such as Asia, sub-Saharan Africa, Eastern Europe, Russia, and Latin America
- Residents and employees of high-risk congregate settings, such as correctional institutions, homeless shelters, nursing homes, mental institutions, and other long-term residential settings
- Health care workers in high-risk settings
- Health care workers with unprotected exposure to a patient with tuberculosis disease before the disease is identified and airborne precautions have been implemented
- Medically underserved, low-income populations as defined locally
- High-risk racial or ethnic minority populations, defined locally as having an increased prevalence of tuberculosis
- Infants, children, and adolescents exposed to people in a high-risk category
- Elderly persons
- Those who inject illicit drugs and any other high-risk substance users as defined locally

When a person has become infected with *M. tuberculosis* there is a greater risk of developing tuberculosis disease if he or she is included in one of the following groups[6]:
- Those with HIV infection
- Persons who were recently infected (within the past two years), particularly those with infants and very young children
- Persons who have a medical condition that is known to increase the risk for disease if infection occurs, including those with the following:
  - Diabetes mellitus
  - Silicosis
  - Prolonged corticosteroid therapy or other immunosuppressive therapy
  - Cancer of the head and neck
  - Hematologic and reticuloendothelial diseases
  - End-state renal disease
  - Intestinal bypass or gastrectomy

– Low body weight
- Persons who inject illicit drugs; also others who use high-risk illicit substances
- Those who have a history of inadequately treated tuberculosis

Patients with active tuberculosis disease who have a higher likelihood of being infectious are those with the following[6]:
- Presence of cough
- Cavitation on chest radiograph
- A positive acid-fast bacilli (AFB) sputum smear
- Respiratory tract disease with involvement of the larynx (substantially infectious)
- Respiratory tract disease with involvement of the lung or pleura (exclusively pleural involvement is less infectious)
- Failure to cover the mouth and nose when coughing
- Incorrect, lack of, or short duration of antituberculosis treatment
- Undergoing cough-inducing or aerosol-generating procedures (for example, bronchoscopy, sputum induction, and administration of aerosolized mediations)

Acid-Fast Bacilli (AFB) Examination
A laboratory test that involves microscopic examination of a stained smear of a patient specimen (usually sputum) to determine if mycobacteria are present. A presumptive diagnosis of pulmonary tuberculosis (TB) can be made with a positive AFB sputum smear result; however, approximately 50% of patients with TB disease of the lungs have negative AFB sputum smear results. The diagnosis of TB disease is usually not confirmed until *Mycobacterium tuberculosis* is identified in culture (*see* Glossary) or by positive nucleic acid amplification test result.

There are also some environmental factors in health care and other settings that increase the risk of transmitting tuberculosis. These include the following:
- Exposure to *M. tuberculosis* in small, enclosed spaces
- Inadequate ventilation that will fail to dilute or remove infectious droplet nuclei
- Recirculation of air containing infectious material
- Failure to adequately clean and disinfect medical devices and equipment
- Handling specimens improperly

Droplet Nuclei
Microscopic particles produced when a person coughs, sneezes, shouts, or sings. These particles can remain suspended in the air for prolonged periods and can be carried on normal air currents in a room and beyond to adjacent spaces or areas receiving exhaust air.

Drug-Resistant Tuberculosis

There are two types of drug resistance: primary resistance and secondary (acquired) resistance. *Primary resistance* occurs when individuals are infected with resistant organisms. *Secondary (acquired) resistance* develops during tuberculosis therapy for one of the two following reasons:

1. The patient was treated with an inadequate therapeutic regimen.
2. The patient did not take the prescribed regimen properly.

Drug-resistant tuberculosis is transmitted by the same process as tuberculosis that is susceptible to drugs.

An increase in MDR strains of *M. tuberculosis* is a growing concern in the United States and throughout the world. MDR-TB is defined as tuberculosis that is resistant to at least two first-line therapies (isoniazid and rifampin). The CDC reports that the number of persons with MDR-TB increased 13.3% in the United States from 2003 to 2004. This was the largest single-year increase in MDR-TB since 1993.

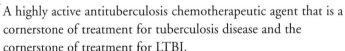

Isoniazid
A highly active antituberculosis chemotherapeutic agent that is a cornerstone of treatment for tuberculosis disease and the cornerstone of treatment for LTBI.

Rifampin
A highly active antituberculosis chemotherapeutic agent that is a cornerstone of treatment for tuberculosis disease.

Of concern is also the fact that MDR-TB tends to be more common in non–U.S.-born persons.

An escalation of drug resistance is the emergence of XDR-TB. XDR-TB is defined as tuberculosis that is resistant to at least two main first-line drugs and, in addition, to three or more of the six classes of second-line drugs. A survey of a worldwide laboratory network conducted from 2000 to 2004 found that isolates tested for 2% of tuberculosis patients met the criteria for XDR-TB. During the five years of this study, XDR-TB increased from 5% of MDR-TB patients in 2000 to 6.5% in 2004 (excluding South Korea). In the industrialized nations (including the United States), XDR-TB increased from 3% to 11% of MDR-TB cases. XDR-TB is virtually untreatable with available drugs and is widely distributed geographically, including in the United States.

The concerns about MDR-TB and XDR-TB emphasize the need for early identification of persons with LTBI and tuberculosis disease, as well as of the contacts of persons with active disease. They also underscore a major reason that every effort should be made to assure that appropriate therapy is implemented and completed. The directly observed therapy approach has had success in monitoring patients and assuring compliance with completing the entire regimen.[7] (For more information on treating patients with drug-resistant tuberculosis, *see* Chapter 2.) The CDC and other agencies involved in the endeavor to eradicate tuberculosis in the United States realize that without the worldwide effort, efforts here would be futile. Therefore, there is truly a cooperative strategy to address these multiple problems internationally.

Summation of the CDC's 2005 Guidelines

The purpose of the CDC's "Guidelines for Preventing the Transmission of *Mycobacterium tuberculosis* in Health-Care Settings, 2005," is to do the following[8]:

• Update and replace the 1994 *M. tuberculosis* infection control guidelines
• Further reduce the threat to health care workers
• Expand the guidelines to nontraditional settings
• Simplify procedures for risk assessment
• Promote vigilance and expertise needed to prevent tuberculosis resurgence

Following is an overview of the guidelines, as well as the changes that have been made and how they impact various health care settings.

Changes in the Guidelines

The changes that appear in the 2005 recommendations were made to reflect the shifts in the epidemiology of tuberculosis and advances in the scientific community's understanding of the disease, as well as changes in clinical practice that have taken place in the United States since the previous document was issued. In particular, the report emphasizes actions that organizations and health care workers can take to maintain the momentum and keep up the levels of expertise needed to prevent another resurgence of the disease and to eliminate the lingering threat to caregivers, which comes primarily from those with unsuspected and undiagnosed infectious tuberculosis disease.

The changes are summarized as follows:
- The risk assessment process has additional aspects of infection control.
- The term *tuberculin skin tests* (TSTs) is used instead of *purified protein derivative.*
- A new blood assay for *M. tuberculosis* (BAMT) has been approved by the U.S. Food and Drug Administration for cell-mediated reactivity and may be used instead of TST in tuberculosis screening programs for health care workers.
- The frequency of tuberculosis screening for health care workers has been decreased in various settings, and the criteria for determination of screening frequency have been changed.
- The scope of settings in which the guidelines apply has been broadened to include laboratories and additional outpatient and nontraditional facility-based settings.
- Criteria for serial testing for *M. tuberculosis* infection of health care workers are more clearly defined.
- The guidelines usually apply to an entire health care setting rather than areas within the setting.
- New terms, airborne infection precautions, and airborne infection isolation rooms (AII rooms) are introduced.
- Recommendations for annual respirator training, initial respirator fit testing, and periodic respirator fit testing have been added.

Blood Assay for *Mycobacterium Tuberculosis* (BAMT)
A general term to refer to recently developed in vitro diagnostic tests that assess for the presence of infection with *M. tuberculosis*. This term includes, but is not limited to, IFN–release assays.

Airborne Infection Isolation (AII) Room

A room designed to maintain AII. Formerly called negative pressure isolation room, an AII room is a single-occupancy patient-care room used to isolate persons with suspected or confirmed infectious TB disease. Environmental factors are controlled in AII rooms to minimize the transmission of infectious agents that are usually spread from person to person by droplet nuclei associated with coughing or aerosolization of contaminated fluids. AII rooms should provide negative pressure in the room (so that air flows under the door gap into the room), an airflow rate of 6–12 ACH, and direct exhaust of air from the room to the outside of the building or recirculation of air through a HEPA filter.

- The evidence of the need for respirator fit testing is summarized.
- Information on ultraviolet germicidal irradiation (UVGI) and room-air recirculation units has been expanded.
- Additional information regarding MDR-TB and HIV infection has been included.

Expanded Vigilance in Other Health Care Settings

Whereas the 1994 recommendations were aimed primarily at hospital-based facilities, the 2005 recommendations have been expanded to include a much wider range of care settings, including outpatient and nontraditional facility-based settings such as the following[6]:
- Tuberculosis treatment facilities
- Medical offices
- Ambulatory care facilities
- Dialysis units
- Dental care facilities
- Emergency medical service
- Medical settings in correctional facilities
- Home-based health care and outreach settings
- Long term care settings, including hospice-skilled nursing facilities
- Homeless shelters
- Other settings where tuberculosis patients might be encountered, such as cafeterias, general stores, kitchens, laundry areas, maintenance shops, pharmacies, and law enforcement settings

The type of health care setting and the people it tends to serve can help determine the types of controls that are necessary to prevent the spread of tuberculosis to health care workers and to other patients in the facility. To define how extensive the administrative, environmental, and respiratory controls (discussed in more detail in Chapter 3) need to be in your organization, the following criteria should be used:

1. If your organization or setting provides services to persons who have suspected or confirmed infectious tuberculosis disease, you should have a tuberculosis infection control plan. This would include laboratories and nontraditional facility-based settings.

2. If your organization or setting is one where patients with suspected or confirmed tuberculosis disease are not expected to be encountered, you still need a less extensive tuberculosis infection control program.

Table 1-2, pages 25–26, provides a comparison between the requirements for health care settings that provide services to tuberculosis patients and those that don't expect to encounter tuberculosis patients.

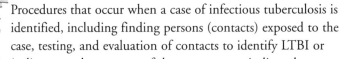

Contact Investigation
Procedures that occur when a case of infectious tuberculosis is identified, including finding persons (contacts) exposed to the case, testing, and evaluation of contacts to identify LTBI or tuberculosis disease, and treatment of these persons, as indicated.

Assessing Risk Classification Under the New Guidelines

In the 1994 guidelines, health care facilities were required to assess and classify risk as *minimal, very low, low, intermediate,* or *high.* The new risk classifications are simplified as *low, medium,* or *potential ongoing transmission.*

The purpose of the risk assessment is to determine the need for a tuberculosis screening program for health care workers and the frequency of screening, which in some cases has been modified from the previous guidelines. A risk assessment is generally determined for the entire setting. However, in complex health care organizations, it is possible to specify separate risk classifications for specific areas. Tuberculosis screenings for health care workers are covered in more detail in Chapter 3.

Table 1-2. Comparison of Program Requirements Based on Whether Tuberculosis Patients Are Likely to Be Encountered

Program Element	Provides Services to Tuberculosis Patients	Tuberculosis Patients Not Expected to Be Encountered
Responsibility for program	Responsibility assigned to a person or group with expertise in LTBI and tuberculosis disease, infection control, and occupational health. Must have the support and authority to conduct a tuberculosis risk assessment, implement and enforce tuberculosis infection control policies, and ensure recommended training and education for health care workers.	Responsibility assigned to appropriate personnel
Tuberculosis infection control plan	Plan must outline a protocol for the prompt recognition and initiation of airborne precautions for persons with suspected or confirmed tuberculosis disease. Plan must be updated annually.	Plan must outline a protocol for the prompt recognition and transfer of persons with suspected or confirmed tuberculosis disease to another health care setting or facility. Plan should include procedures for separation of these persons from other persons in the setting until they are transferred. Evaluate the plan annually.
Problem evaluation for cases of suspected or confirmed tuberculosis disease when not readily recognized or properly isolated	Conduct a problem evaluation each time a case is not promptly recognized, and airborne precautions not initiated, or if administrative, environmental, or respiratory protection controls fail.	Conduct evaluation if a case is not promptly recognized, separated from others, and transferred.

(continued)

Table 1-2. Comparison of Program Requirements Based on Whether Tuberculosis Patients Are Likely to Be Encountered, *continued*

Program Element	Provides Services to Tuberculosis Patients	Tuberculosis Patients Not Expected to Be Encountered
Contact investigation in collaboration with local or state health department	Perform a contact investigation if health care–associated transmission of tuberculosis is suspected. Implement and monitor corrective actions.	Investigate if health care–associated transmission of tuberculosis is suspected.
Collaboration with local or state health department to develop administrative controls	Administrative controls to consist of the following: • The risk assessment • Written tuberculosis infection control plan • Management of patients with suspected or confirmed tuberculosis • Training and education of health care workers • Problem evaluation • Coordination	Administrative controls to consist of the following: • Risk assessment • Written tuberculosis infection control plan
Environmental controls	Implement and maintain environmental controls, including All rooms.	
Respiratory-protection program	Implement a respiratory-protection program.	
Training and Education	Perform initial and ongoing training and education of health care workers.	
Plan for accepting transferred patients	Develop a plan for accepting patients who have suspected or confirmed tuberculosis disease if they are transferred from another setting.	

Source: Centers for Disease Control and Prevention: Guidelines for preventing the transmission of *Mycobacterium tuberculosis* in health-care settings, 2005. *MMWR Recomm Rep* 54:1–147, Dec. 30, 2005.

Low Risk

This classification is for settings where persons with tuberculosis disease are not expected to be encountered, and, as a result, exposure to *M. tuberculosis* is unlikely. The classification may also be applied to health care workers who will never be exposed to persons with tuberculosis disease or to clinical specimens that could contain *M. tuberculosis.*

Medium Risk

The medium risk classification is to be used in settings where health care workers will or will possibly be exposed to persons with tuberculosis disease or specimens that might contain *M. tuberculosis.*

Potential Ongoing Transmission

This is a temporary classification that is applied to any setting or group of health care workers if there is evidence to suggest that person-to-person transmission of *M. tuberculosis* has occurred in the setting during the preceding year.

In its 2005 recommendations, the CDC provides a worksheet for assisting organizations in determining risk. Table 1-3, pages 28–29, lists factors that should be addressed when determining the risk classification for your setting.

Settings that serve communities with a high incidence of tuberculosis disease or that treat populations at high risk might need to be classified as medium risk even if they meet the low-risk criteria.

New Guidelines for Screening of Health Care Workers

After the risk assessment has been performed and the relative risk of exposure for various groups of health care workers determined, the organization can implement or revise an employee surveillance program according to the new guidelines. One of the new additions to the 2005 recommendations is the approval of one blood assay for *M. tuberculosis* that may be used in place of the TST. In addition, for health care workers who work in low-risk settings and who have not been exposed to tuberculosis patients, the requirement to continue serial testing after a negative baseline test has been dropped. Table 1-4, page 30, gives the new recommendations for screening of health care workers. Chapter 3 includes a table to help you determine the risk level for your facility.

Table 1-3. Factors for Consideration When Performing a Risk Assessment

Factors for Consideration	Settings Where Patients with Suspected or Confirmed Tuberculosis Disease Are Expected to Be Encountered	Settings Where Patients with Suspected or Confirmed Tuberculosis Disease Are NOT Expected to Be Encountered
Review the community profile of tuberculosis disease with state or local health department.	X	X
Consult local or state tuberculosis control program to obtain epidemiologic surveillance data as it relates to your setting.	X	X
Review the number of patients with suspected or confirmed tuberculosis disease in the setting during the last five years or longer.	X	
Determine if patients with unrecognized tuberculosis disease have been admitted to or were encountered in the last five years.	X	X
Determine which health care workers need to be included in a screening program and the frequency of screening based on risk classification.	X	Determine if any health care workers need to be included in the tuberculosis screening program.
Process for the prompt recognition and evaluation of suspected episodes of health care–associated transmission of *M. tuberculosis*.	X	Document procedures that address this issue.

(continued)

Table 1-3. Factors for Consideration When Performing a Risk Assessment, *continued*

Factors for Consideration	Settings Where Patients with Suspected or Confirmed Tuberculosis Disease Are Expected to Be Encountered	Settings Where Patients with Suspected or Confirmed Tuberculosis Disease Are NOT Expected to Be Encountered
Identify areas in the setting with an increased risk of the above and target them for improved tuberculosis infection controls.	X	
Assess the number of AII rooms needed for the setting.	X	
Determine the types of environmental controls in place and needed.	X	X
Determine which health care workers need to be included in the respiratory protection program.	X	
Conduct periodic reassessments annually to ensure proper implementation of the plan and prompt detection of suspected tuberculosis cases, along with appropriate responses.	X	X
Recognize and correct lapses in infection control.	X	X

Source: Centers for Disease Control and Prevention: Guidelines for preventing the transmission of *Mycobacterium tuberculosis* in health-care settings, 2005. *MMWR Recomm Rep* 54:1–147, Dec. 30, 2005.

Table 1-4. Screening Frequency for Health Care Workers

Screening Frequency	Low Risk	Medium Risk	Potential Ongoing Transmission
Baseline two-step TST or one BAMT for all health care workers upon hire	Yes	Yes	Yes
Serial TST or BAMT screening of health care workers	No	Every 12 months	As needed in the investigation of potential ongoing transmission; may need to be performed every 8–10 weeks until lapses in infection control have been corrected.
Health care workers with a baseline positive or newly positive test result or documentation of treatment for LTBI or tuberculosis disease should have a chest radiograph to exclude tuberculosis disease.	Yes	Yes	Yes
TST or BAMT for health care workers upon unprotected exposure to *M. tuberculosis:* Perform a contact investigation (administer one TST as soon as possible at the time of exposure, and if the TST result is negative, perform another TST 8–10 weeks after the end of the exposure).	Yes	Yes	Yes

Source: Centers for Disease Control and Prevention: Guidelines for preventing the transmission of *Mycobacterium tuberculosis* in health-care settings, 2005. *MMWR Recomm Rep* 54:1–147, Dec. 30, 2005.

A TST conversion is considered to be an increase equal to or greater than 10 mm in the size of the TST indurations in a two-year period for the following:

1. A health care worker with a documented negative baseline two-step TST

   or

2. A person who is not a health care worker with a negative TST result within two years

The following are two calculations important in maintaining vigilance regarding infection control practices and the need for additional safeguards:

- Conversion rates for employees, which can indicate a review of infection control practices if they rise above the baseline
- Reassessment of the risk for the setting, particularly if the initial risk was low and serial testing of employees is not performed

Clinical Advancements

Because of increased concerns about concurrent HIV and tuberculosis, as well as MDR organisms, there has been more emphasis on developing new tests to expedite the identification of patients with infectious tuberculosis disease, as well as isolation and treatment. In fact, in the WHO's *The Global Plan to Stop TB 2006–2015,* two of the objectives are the following:

- By 2010, diagnostic tests at the point of care will allow rapid, sensitive, and inexpensive detection of active tuberculosis. By 2012, a diagnostic toolbox will accurately identify people with LTBI and those at high risk of progression to the disease.
- By 2015, a new, safe, effective, and affordable test will be available with potential for a significant impact on tuberculosis control in later years.

Some of the clinical advancements currently under way in the United States include the following:

- The new blood test for screening for LTBI. Although only one blood test is currently approved, others are undergoing trials, and may be available in the near future.
- An improved vaccine. There are attempts to develop such a vaccine, though it has not yet been accomplished.
- The development of rapid NAA tests allow for one-day identification of *M. tuberculosis.* However, these tests should not replace culture and drug-susceptibility testing in patients with suspected tuberculosis disease. Mixed mycobacterial infection may obscure the identification of *M. tuberculosis* during laboratory testing. The specific bacterial identification can be determined by the use of DNA probes. In addition, colony morphology examination on solid culture media can be useful in identifying the organism. Drug susceptibility tests need to be performed on all initial isolates to assist in identifying the correct treatment regimen. The test is also useful in identifying MDR organisms.

Other Tuberculosis Guidelines and Regulations

The Joint Commission Standards for Surveillance, Prevention, and Control of Infection readily crosswalk with the CDC's "Guidelines for Preventing the Transmission of *Mycobacterium tuberculosis* in Health-Care Facilities, 2005." Requirements associated with these standards are discussed in more detail in Chapter 3.

Agencies other than the CDC that have defined guidelines or regulations related to tuberculosis include the National Institute for Occupational Safety and Health (NIOSH), the Occupational Safety and Health Administration (OSHA), and various state departments of health. The NIOSH is a division of the CDC, and its purpose is to provide research, information, education, and training in the area of occupational safety and health. OSHA is the agency required to set and enforce standards to improve occupational safety and health. Therefore, the NIOSH provides educational materials for topics such as "Tuberculosis Respiratory Protection," and provides reports on its research on the most effective respirators and the use of UVGI light in destroying *M. tuberculosis,* for example. OSHA, however, has a directive that provides uniform inspection procedures and guidelines to be followed when conducting inspections and issuing citations under Section 5(a)(1) of the Occupational Safety and Health (OSH) Act and pertinent standards for employees who are occupationally exposed to tuberculosis.[9] The agency also has regulatory requirements regarding recording and reporting occupational illnesses and tuberculosis and respiratory protection, including requirements for respirators, fit testing, a written program, training for staff, and record keeping (*see* Sidebar 1-2, page 33, for more information).

In addition, states may have very specific regulations that are more stringent than the CDC guidelines or OSHA regulations. It is important that each health care setting be aware of any specific state or local regulations not included in the CDC guidelines or OSHA regulations.

Sidebar 1-2.
Occupational Safety and Health Administration's Tuberculosis Policy

Employers must comply with the provisions of the following requirements whenever an employee may be occupationally exposed to tuberculosis.

Section 5(a)(1)—General Duty Clause and Executive Order 12196, Section 1-201(a) for Federal Facilities

Section 5(a)(1) of the OSH Act states: "Each employer shall furnish to each of his employees employment and a place of employment which are free from recognized hazards that are causing or are likely to cause death or serious physical harm to his employees." OSHA will issue citations to employers with employees working in one of the workplaces where the CDC has identified workers as having a higher incidence of tuberculosis infection than the general population, when the employees are not provided appropriate protection and have tuberculosis exposure.

29 CFR 1910.134—Respiratory Protection

The primary means to control occupational diseases caused by breathing contaminated air is through the use of feasible engineering controls such as enclosures, confinement of operations, ventilation, or substitution of less toxic materials. When these controls are not feasible, or while they are being instituted, appropriate respirators shall be used.

29 CFR 1910.145—Accident Prevention Signs and Tags

A warning or a message referring one to the nursing station for instruction shall be posted outside the respiratory isolation or treatment room. A signal word or biological hazard symbol must be presented, as well as a major message. Employers are also required to use biological hazard tags on air transport components to identify to employees the tuberculosis hazards associated with working on air systems that transport contaminated air.

29 CFR 1910.1020—Access to Employee Exposure and Medical Records

Records concerning employee exposure to tuberculosis, tuberculosis skin test results, and medical evaluations and treatments are employee medical records and should be treated as such.

Source: Occupational Safety and Health Administration: *Overview of Enforcement for Occupational Exposure to Tuberculosis*. http://www.osha.gov/dcsp/ote/trng-materials/tuberculosis/tbpresent/index.html (accessed Sep. 13, 2007).

References

1. Centers for Disease Control and Prevention (CDC): *CDC's Response to Ending Neglect: The Elimination of Tuberculosis in the United States.* Atlanta: U.S. Department of Health and Human Services, CDC, 2002.

2. World Health Organization: The Global Plan to Stop TB 2006–2015. http://www.who.int/tb/features_archive/global_plan_to_stop_tb/en/index.html (accessed Jul. 11, 2007).

3. Cantwell M.F., et al.: Epidemiology of tuberculosis in the United States, 1985 through 1992. *JAMA* 272:535–539, Aug. 17, 1994.

4. Centers for Disease Control and Prevention: *Reported Tuberculosis in the United States 2005.* http://www.cdc.gov/tb/surv/surv2005/ (accessed Oct. 2, 2007).

5. Centers for Disease Control and Prevention (CDC): *Core Curriculum on Tuberculosis: What the Clinician Should Know,* 4th ed. Atlanta: CDC, 2000.

6. Centers for Disease Control and Prevention: Guidelines for preventing the transmission of *Mycobacterium tuberculosis* in health-care settings, 2005. *MMWR Recomm Rep* 54:1–147, Dec. 30, 2005.

7. Centers for Disease Control and Prevention: Emergence of *Mycobacterium tuberculosis* with extensive resistance to second-line drugs—Worldwide, 2000–2004. *MMWR Morb Mortal Wkly Rep* 55:301–305, Mar. 24, 2006.

8. Centers for Disease Control and Prevention: *Slide Set—Guidelines for Preventing the Transmission of* M. tuberculosis *in Health-Care Settings, 2005.* http://www.cdc.gov/tb/pubs/slidesets/InfectionGuidelines/default.htm (accessed Oct. 2, 2007).

9. Occupational Safety and Health Administration: *CPL 02-00-106–CPL 2.106–Enforcement Procedures and Scheduling for Occupational Exposure to Tuberculosis.* http://www.osha.gov/pls/oshaweb/owadisp.show_document?p_table=DIRECTIVES&p_id=1586 (accessed Oct. 2, 2007).

Chapter 2

Early Identification and Isolation of Infectious Individuals

The experts agree: Early diagnosis, isolation, and treatment of persons with tuberculosis are among the most important steps in arresting the disease. However, the need to diagnose the disease as quickly as possible is complicated in the United States by the very success of the public health efforts in reducing the actual number of tuberculosis cases and outbreaks. There are very real concerns that as the incidence of the disease declines, health care workers will have less expertise in identifying the clinical symptoms that are indicative of tuberculosis.

Identifying Patients with Tuberculosis

It is extremely important to identify persons with *Mycobacterium tuberculosis* as quickly as possible, but this process requires a stance of continued vigilance and awareness on the part of health care professionals. In some organizations, it is a rare event to have an emergency or other ambulatory patient present with tuberculosis. In these organizations, the challenge is to remain alert to tuberculosis as a possible diagnosis, along with that of other diseases.

To properly identify patients, family, and health care workers who may have tuberculosis, clinicians need to maintain an awareness of the following factors:
- Symptoms of active pulmonary tuberculosis
- Identification of elements that place persons at a higher risk for exposure to and infection with *M. tuberculosis*
- Unique aspects of the disease and means of transmission in different settings
- Tests required to diagnose and confirm successful treatment of tuberculosis
- Required isolation of patients with active pulmonary tuberculosis, along with protective measures for anyone coming in contact with these patients, their airspace, or specimens of infected persons, including health care workers, family members, and others in close contact with an infectious individual prior to diagnosis

The need to enforce this awareness requires initial training and education programs and ongoing periodic updates for health care professional staff. More details about training and education for health care workers can be found in Chapter 4.

Health care workers must also be aware that several types of tuberculosis infection can occur. Tuberculosis is a chronic infection that usually infects the lungs, but may enter an individual's bloodstream and infect other areas in the body, such as lymph nodes, bones, joints, and kidneys. In addition, only a small percentage of persons infected with tuberculosis will go on to develop the active disease during their lifetime. Most people infected with *M. tuberculosis* have latent tuberculosis infection (LTBI). When a person has contracted LTBI, the risk for progression to tuberculosis disease varies. However, it is still important to try to identify those with LTBI because there is a chance that the infection will progress to infectious tuberculosis disease when the individual's immune system becomes compromised from another disease or as the person becomes older.

Risk Factors for Tuberculosis

Knowing the factors that increase tuberculosis risk is one tool for identifying people with the infection. The people who are at the highest risk for exposure to, and therefore infection with, *M. tuberculosis* are the following:

- Close contacts of the infected individual, such as family, friends, or those who share living space
- Residents and staff of high-risk settings, such as long term care or correctional facilities
- Non–U.S.-born people from foreign countries with a high tuberculosis incidence
- Health care workers serving high-risk clients or those unknowingly exposed to tuberculosis patients
- Low-income, medically underserved groups
- Locally defined high-risk groups
- Children exposed to high-risk adults

LTBI progresses to tuberculosis in a small number of individuals soon after infection. It also progresses for some persons with untreated LTBI some time during their lifetime, and to persons with human immunodeficiency virus (HIV)/acquired immune deficiency syndrome (AIDS) and untreated LTBI. Therefore, those individuals who are at highest risk for progressing to tuberculosis disease are the following:

- Those who have a coinfection of HIV and *M. tuberculosis.* More than a quarter of tuberculosis cases in the United States appear attributable to HIV infection, underscoring the importance of both tuberculosis and HIV/AIDS treatment programs.[1]
- Persons with recent infection within the last two years; 5% of these individuals will progress to active tuberculosis disease.
- Children under 4 years of age
- Those with conditions of compromised immunity
- Persons with a history of untreated or poorly treated tuberculosis

Transmission of tuberculosis is most likely to result from the following types of patients:
- Those with unsuspected pulmonary tuberculosis disease who are not receiving antituberculosis treatment
- Those with diagnosed tuberculosis disease who are receiving inadequate therapy
- Those with diagnosed tuberculosis disease who are early in the course of therapy that will be effective

There is a correlation between the infectiousness of a patient's tuberculosis and the number of organisms he or she expels into the air, and may be related to the following[2]:
- The presence of a cough that lasts for a long period of time (more than three weeks)
- Presence of cavitation on the chest radiograph
- Positive sputum smear acid-fast bacilli (AFB) results
- Respiratory tract disease with involvement of the lungs or airways, including the larynx
- Failure to cover the mouth and nose when coughing
- A lack of correct or incorrectly short duration of treatment for tuberculosis
- Undergoing cough-inducing or aerosol-producing procedures

Some of the environmental factors that increase the risk for infectiousness transmission include the following:
- Poor or no ventilation, particularly with overcrowding. Exposure in confined systems with little ventilation or no ventilation poses a significant risk for transmission of tuberculosis. When contact occurs outdoors, tuberculosis bacilli expelled from the respiratory tract are quickly dispersed and rendered harmless by sunlight.
- Hospital areas where cough-induction or aerosol-producing procedures are performed. The risk of transmission in these areas is increased unless environmental controls (for example, negative ventilation) are implemented.

In health care settings, there is an increased risk for health care workers to become infected, particularly from undiagnosed patients. There is also a risk that patients will become infected from a health care worker who has not been diagnosed or who has not undergone therapy. Chapter 3 provides more information on preventing transmission of the disease between patients and health care workers.

Diagnosis

An essential element in eliminating tuberculosis is early diagnosis and follow-up treatment, as well as adequate contact investigation to identify others who may have become infected by contact with the primary individual. Ongoing advances in test methods continue to progress and have the ability to help expedite the testing process. However, the first consideration is identifying an individual as being at risk and either having symptoms of active disease or having the potential for LTBI.

This challenge is compounded by the very success in the decrease of incidence of tuberculosis in the United States and other countries. This means that health care professionals see fewer patients with tuberculosis and, therefore, have less experience with diagnosing the disease. Therefore, it is imperative that clinicians remain alert for the possibility of tuberculosis when examining patients with potential symptoms of the illness that represent active tuberculosis or LTBI. Health care professionals need to remain aware of the risk factors for tuberculosis, as well as the signs and symptoms.[3] For more on education and training, *see* Chapter 4 of this book.

Assessing Symptoms

The symptoms of pulmonary and extrapulmonary tuberculosis may differ, but some symptoms are common to both. Patients do not usually present with all or even most of the following symptoms, and care providers should be suspicious if patients have been experiencing three or more of the following symptoms for three or more weeks, including a dry or productive prolonged cough (duration equal to or greater than three weeks), chest pain, shortness of breath, or hemoptysis (coughing up blood or blood-tinged sputum).

When a person presents in a health care setting with these symptoms, tuberculosis should be a primary consideration.[4]

The following are systemic or general symptoms of tuberculosis:
- Fever
- Chills
- Night sweats
- Loss of appetite
- Unintended weight loss
- Fatigue
- Localized pain and/or swelling (depending on the site of the disease)

For health care workers who are familiar with tuberculosis and its symptoms, the disease can still be difficult to diagnose. Most patients do not present with a majority of the above symptoms. In fact, patients usually present with only a few symptoms. For example, in one study of tuberculosis patients in the emergency department, cough was present in only 64% of the cases and was the chief complaint in less than 20% of the cases.[5] In addition, many of the symptoms of tuberculosis are also symptoms of other common ailments, such as cold and flu. The clinician should be suspicious if the patient has experienced three or more of the symptoms for three or more weeks.

Because tuberculosis progresses differently in children it is more difficult to diagnose. Children are usually unable to cough hard enough to produce sputum for testing, and radiograph changes are less well defined.

One half of all patients with tuberculosis disease can present with negative sputum smears.[6] In the later stages of HIV infection, patients are likely to present with less definable symptoms than the norm, making identification more challenging, and finally, in private hospitals where tuberculosis disease is seldom seen, the diagnosis is more likely to be missed.[7]

Physical Examination
A physical examination is always a vital component of diagnosing any disease. With tuberculosis, the examinations do not, in and of themselves, confirm or disprove tuberculosis. However, examinations can provide necessary information about an individual's overall health and conditions that could affect how tuberculosis would be treated.

Testing

There are several tests used to diagnose tuberculosis, including the following:
- Tuberculin skin testing
- Blood assay for detection of *M. tuberculosis*
- Chest radiograph
- Diagnostic microbiology testing:
  - Acid-fast stained smears
  - Sputum culture with susceptibility testing
  - Nucleic acid probes and amplification tests

Tuberculin Skin Testing

The tuberculin skin test (TST), formerly known as the purified protein derivative (PPD) or the Mantoux method, has traditionally been used to screen individuals who are not ill but may be infected with *M. tuberculosis*—for example, someone who may have LTBI (TST can be used to test patients presenting with tuberculosis symptoms as well).

TST is primarily used in the following situations:
1. In contact investigations to test close contacts of people who have active tuberculosis disease
2. As part of targeted testing activities for various groups of people who are at high risk for tuberculosis, such as health care workers who serve high-risk clients, residents and employees of correctional facilities, and non–U.S.-born people from areas that have a high tuberculosis incidence
3. In routine wellness examinations, most often for children and for young adults preparing for school (for example, many schools require the TST as part of the physical examination given to children before beginning kindergarten)

The TST has several steps that require adequate and appropriate training for administration, as well as for reading it. These steps can lead to erroneous results if not performed properly. Therefore, training to perform and read the test must be stringent, and there should be quality controls of test performance. Patients should not be allowed to read their own TST results; rather, they must return to their care provider to have the results read by a trained health care worker. The following are the critical steps that must be properly performed:
1. The injection of 0.1 mL of PPD into the surface of the forearm. If the patient has been infected with *M. tuberculosis,* the PPD will cause a reaction that results in a round, raised area on the skin, known as an induration.

2. Reading of the test results:
   a. Within the defined timeframe (48 to 72 hours after the injection)
   b. Reading the induration (the raised area) and not the area of redness
   c. Measuring the induration in millimeters against a standardized measuring device
3. Interpreting the results correctly for the intended purpose

Targeted tuberculin testing is a component of tuberculosis control used to identify persons at high risk for developing tuberculosis who would benefit from treatment of LTBI. Interpretation of targeted testing results requires knowledge of each person's risk for being infected with *M. tuberculosis.* Table 2-1, page 42, provides positive result readings for specified groups. Sidebar 2-1, pages 43–47, is a quick quiz you can use to see how much you know about the diagnosis of tuberculosis.

On the other hand, when the TST is used as part of a tuberculosis infection control program, different interpretation criteria are used. When screening health care workers, the interpretation of TST results is performed in two steps. The first step is an interpretation by standard criteria, and the second step is the interpretation by individualized criteria to determine the need for treatment of LTBI (*see* Table 2-2, page 48).

Although it is the most commonly used tuberculosis test, TST is not 100% accurate. Challenges that can prevent an exact diagnosis through TST are discussed in the next sections.

Anergy
Even if the skin test reaction is negative, a diagnosis of tuberculosis infection or disease cannot be completely ruled out. In immunosuppressed individuals, reactions of delayed-type hypersensitivity can decrease or completely disappear. This phenomenon, called anergy, should be considered in persons with the following conditions:
- HIV infection
- Severe or febrile illness
- Overwhelming tuberculosis disease
- Viral infections
- Live virus vaccinations
- Immunosuppressive therapy

Anergy can be detected by giving at least two other delayed-type hypersensitivity antigens by the Mantoux method. However, the lack of standardization and outcome

Table 2-1. Positive Result Readings

Group A	Group B	Group C
Induration Reading Equal to or Greater Than 5 mm	**Induration Reading Equal to or Greater Than 10 mm**	**Induration Reading Equal to or Greater Than 15 mm**
Classified as positive for the following: • HIV–positive persons • Recent contacts of tuberculosis case • Persons with fibrotic changes on chest radiograph consistent with old healed tuberculosis • Patients with organ transplants or other immunosuppressed patients	Classified as positive for persons not meeting the criteria in Group A but with other risk factors for tuberculosis, such as the following: • Recent arrivals (last five years) from high-incidence countries • Injection drug users • Residents and employees of high-risk congregate settings • Mycobacteriology laboratory personnel • Persons with clinical conditions that place them at high risk • Children less than 4 years of age, or children and adolescents exposed to	Classified as positive for persons with no known risk factors for tuberculosis

Source: Centers for Disease Control and Prevention: *BCG Vaccine.* http://www.cdc.gov/tb/pubs/tbfactsheets/BCG.htm (accessed Jul. 30, 2007).

data have led to a conclusion that anergy testing should no longer be routinely used in TST programs for HIV–positive persons in the United States.

False Positives and Negatives

In some people who are infected with *M. tuberculosis,* a skin test given many years after infection may produce a negative result. However, this skin test may stimulate a person's ability to react to tuberculin, causing a positive reaction to subsequent tests; this boosted reaction may be misinterpreted as a new infection. This phenomenon may occur in patients of any age, but its frequency increases with age. Boosted reactions may also occur in people infected with nontuberculous mycobacteria or in those who have had a prior Bacille Calmette-Guérin (BCG) vaccination.

Sidebar 2-1.
Quiz Yourself—Diagnosis of Tuberculosis

1. A 30-year-old man visits the health department for a TST because he is required to have one before starting his new job. He has a positive reaction to the TST. He has no symptoms of tuberculosis and his chest x-ray findings are normal.
   - Should this be considered a case of tuberculosis?
     The man described above has tuberculosis infection, but he has no evidence of tuberculosis disease. Therefore, this is not a case of tuberculosis.
   - Should this man be considered infectious?
     No, he should not be considered infectious. This man has tuberculosis infection, not tuberculosis disease. People with tuberculosis infection and no evidence of tuberculosis disease are not infectious. (Note that sputum tests were not done. Sputum tests are not necessary when a person has no symptoms of tuberculosis and has normal chest x-ray findings. However, if they had been done, we would expect them to be negative.)

2. A 45-year-old woman is referred to the local health department by her private physician because she was found to have tuberculosis infection. She is an obese woman who has high blood pressure and heart problems. Upon further questioning, she reports that she has injected illicit drugs in the past but has never been tested for HIV infection.
   - What conditions does this woman have that increase the risk that she will develop tuberculosis disease?
     One condition is injection of illicit drugs, which increases the risk that tuberculosis infection will progress to tuberculosis disease. Another possible condition is HIV infection. This woman is at risk for HIV infection, which is the strongest known risk factor for developing tuberculosis disease. This woman should undergo HIV counseling and testing. Obesity, high blood pressure, and heart problems are NOT risk factors for tuberculosis disease.

3. Which of the following patients have a positive tuberculin skin test reaction?
   a. Mr. West, 36 years old, HIV infected, 8 mm of induration
   b. Ms. Hernandez, 26 years old, native of Mexico, 7 mm of induration

(continued)

Sidebar 2-1.
Quiz Yourself—Diagnosis of Tuberculosis, *continued*

  c. Ms. Jones, 56 years old, has diabetes, 12 mm of induration
  d. Mr. Sung, 79 years old, resident of a nursing home, 11 mm of induration
  e. Mr. Williams, 21 years old, no risk factors, 13 mm of induration
  f. Ms. Marcos, 42 years old, chest x-ray findings suggestive of previous tuberculosis, 6 mm of induration
  g. Ms. Rayle, 50 years old, husband has pulmonary tuberculosis, 9 mm of induration

Answers: a, c, d, f, g

4. A 30-year-old man who recently immigrated from India is given a TST and is found to have 14 millimeters of induration. He reports that he was vaccinated with BCG as a child. He also says that his wife was treated for pulmonary tuberculosis disease last year.
 • Can you tell for sure whether this man has tuberculosis infection?
   No. This man does have a positive reaction to the TST (10 or more millimeters is considered a positive reaction for a non–U.S.-born person from a high-incidence country). However, this may be a false positive reaction because he has been vaccinated with BCG.
 • What factors make it more likely that this man's positive reaction is due to tuberculosis infection?
   First, this man has a fairly large reaction (14 mm). Second, he was vaccinated with BCG a long time ago, when he was a child. Third, this man is from an area of the world where tuberculosis is common, so he was probably exposed to tuberculosis in his native country. Therefore, he is presumed to be at increased risk for tuberculosis infection. Fourth, his wife has had pulmonary tuberculosis, which further increases the probability that he has been exposed to tuberculosis.
   Because he has a positive skin test reaction, this man should be further evaluated for tuberculosis disease.

5. Mr. Bell comes to the tuberculosis clinic for a TST. He believes that he has been exposed to tuberculosis, and he knows he is at high risk for tuberculosis

(continued)

Sidebar 2-1.
Quiz Yourself—Diagnosis of Tuberculosis, *continued*

because he is HIV infected. He is given a TST and his reaction is read 48 hours later as 0 millimeters of induration.

- What are three ways to interpret this result?

  There are three possible reasons why Mr. Bell had no reaction to the tuberculin skin test.

  - He may not have tuberculosis infection.
  - He may be anergic (*see* pages 41–42). People who are HIV infected are more likely to be anergic than persons who are not HIV infected. If Mr. Bell is anergic, he would be unable to react to tuberculin even if he did have tuberculosis infection. To determine whether he is anergic, a clinician can test him with two substances other than tuberculin.
  - It may be less than 10 weeks since he was exposed to tuberculosis. After tuberculosis has been transmitted, it takes 2 to 10 weeks before tuberculosis infection can be detected by the TST. Mr. Bell should be retested 10 weeks after he was last exposed to tuberculosis.

6. Ms. Wilson is a 60-year-old nurse. When she started a job at the local hospital, she was given a TST, her first test in 25 years. Her reaction was read 48 hours later as 0 millimeters of induration. Six months later, she was retested as part of the tuberculosis screening program in the unit where she works. Her skin test reaction was read 48 hours later as 11 millimeters of induration.

- What are two ways to interpret this result?

  There are two possible explanations for this result.

  - Ms. Wilson may have been exposed to and infected with *M. tuberculosis* sometime in the six months between her first and second skin tests.
  - Ms. Wilson may be a victim of the booster phenomenon. If Ms. Wilson was infected with *M. tuberculosis* many years ago, her ability to react to tuberculin may have decreased. This would explain why she did not react to the first tuberculin skin test. Then the first tuberculin test may have boosted the ability of her immune system to react to tuberculin. This would explain why she had a positive reaction to the second test,

(continued)

Sidebar 2-1.
Quiz Yourself—Diagnosis of Tuberculosis, *continued*

which was given within a year of the first test. If this scenario is true, Ms. Wilson's positive reaction would not mean that she was recently infected with *M. tuberculosis.*

This problem in interpreting Ms. Wilson's reaction would have been avoided if she had been tested with a two-step procedure when she first joined the hospital. In any event, because she has a positive reaction, Ms. Wilson should be evaluated for tuberculosis disease.

7. Mr. Lee has a cough and other symptoms of tuberculosis disease, and he is evaluated with a chest x-ray. However, he is unable to cough up any sputum on his own for the bacteriologic examination.
   - What should be done?
   If a patient cannot cough up a sputum specimen, other techniques can be used to obtain sputum. First, clinicians can try to obtain an induced sputum sample. If they cannot obtain an induced sputum sample, a bronchoscopy or gastric washing may be done.

8. Ms. Thompson gave three sputum specimens, which were sent to the laboratory for smear examination and culture. The smear results were reported as 4+, 3+, and 4+.
   - What do these results tell you about Ms. Thompson's diagnosis and her infectiousness?
   These results show that Ms. Thompson's sputum specimens contain many acid-fast bacilli (AFB). Because the smears are positive, clinicians should suspect that Ms. Thompson has tuberculosis disease. They should also consider her to be infectious. However, it is possible that these AFB are mycobacteria other than tubercle bacilli. Therefore, the diagnosis of tuberculosis disease cannot be proven until the culture results are available.

9. Mr. Sagoo has symptoms of tuberculosis disease and a cavity on his chest x-ray, but all of his sputum smears are negative for AFB.
   - Does this rule out the diagnosis of pulmonary tuberculosis disease?
   No. *M. tuberculosis* may grow in the cultures even though there was no AFB on the smear. Mr. Sagoo's symptoms and his abnormal chest x-ray suggest that he does have pulmonary tuberculosis disease.

(continued)

Sidebar 2-1.
Quiz Yourself—Diagnosis of Tuberculosis, *continued*

10. In the public health clinic, you see a patient, Ms. Sanchez, who complains of weight loss, fever, and a cough of four weeks' duration. When questioned, she reports that she has been treated for tuberculosis disease in the past and that she occasionally injects heroin.

    • What parts of Ms. Sanchez's medical history lead you to suspect tuberculosis disease?

      Ms. Sanchez has symptoms of tuberculosis disease (weight loss, fever, and a persistent cough). Also, in the past she has been treated for tuberculosis disease. We don't know whether she completed therapy, but until we can prove otherwise, we should assume that she has tuberculosis disease again. Her history of injecting illicit drugs (heroin) is another risk factor for tuberculosis.

    • What diagnostic tests should be done?

      People who have tuberculosis symptoms should be evaluated for tuberculosis disease. Because she has symptoms of pulmonary tuberculosis disease (coughing), Ms. Sanchez should be given a chest x-ray. In addition, a sputum specimen should be collected for smear and culture, and drug susceptibility testing should be done if the culture is positive for *M. tuberculosis*. A TST may be helpful for the diagnosis of tuberculosis, but it is not necessary.

Source: Centers for Disease Control and Prevention: *Self-Study Modules on Tuberculosis.* http://www.cdc.gov/tb/pubs/SSmodules/default.htm. (accessed Jul. 30. 2007).

Two-step testing can help reduce the likelihood that a boosted reaction like this will be misinterpreted as a recent infection. If the reaction to the first test is classified as negative, a second test should be conducted one to three weeks later. A positive reaction to the second test probably represents a boosted reaction; the person should be classified as previously infected and cared for accordingly. If the second test result is negative, the person should be classified as uninfected.

In these patients, a positive result for any subsequent test is likely to represent a new *M. tuberculosis* infection. Two-step testing should be used for the initial skin testing of adults who will be retested periodically, such as health care workers.

Table 2-2. **Test Result Criteria for Health Care Workers**

Testing Type	Baseline	Serial Testing Without Known Exposure	Known Exposure
TST Result Criteria	Induration equal to or greater than 10 mm is considered a positive result in either first or second step of testing.	Increase equal to or greater than 10 mm is considered a positive result (TST conversion).	Induration equal to or greater than 5 mm is considered a positive result for persons who had a baseline test result of 0 mm; an increase equal to or greater than 10 mm is considered a positive result for persons with a negative baseline TST result or previous follow-up screening result equal to or greater than 0 mm.

Source: Centers for Disease Control and Prevention: Guidelines for preventing the transmission of *Mycobacterium tuberculosis* in health-care settings, 2005. *MMWR Recomm Rep* 54:1–147, Dec. 30, 2005.

Because of cross-reactions with other mycobacteria, the specificity of the tuberculin test is reduced when serial skin testing is performed, as compared with the administration of a single test. Thus, serial skin-testing programs tend to overestimate the incidence of new tuberculosis infection in the tested population. Because of this potential for overestimation of new infections, serial skin-testing programs should be targeted to populations at high risk for continued exposure to infectious persons.

Chest Radiography

A posterior-anterior radiograph of the chest is the standard view used to detect chest abnormalities. In pulmonary tuberculosis, lesions may appear anywhere in the lungs, although abnormalities often include upper lobe infiltration, cavitation, and effusion.

Chest radiographs are also indicated to exclude pulmonary tuberculosis disease in those patients being considered for treatment of LTBI. Chest radiographs are usually normal in patients with LTBI, unless there are abnormalities consistent with previous healed tuberculosis disease or other pulmonary conditions.

Although chest radiography is an essential part of the medical evaluation for tuberculosis disease, it cannot be used to confirm tuberculosis disease.

Diagnostic Microbiology Testing
The full complement of microbiological testing includes the following:
- Collection of a proper specimen
- Initial evaluation of a stained smear
- Culture of the specimen and identification techniques
- Susceptibility testing

Centers for Disease Control and Prevention (CDC) guidelines advocate sputum examination for the following persons:
- Anyone suspected of having pulmonary or laryngeal tuberculosis disease
- Persons with chest radiograph findings consistent with tuberculosis disease (current, previous, or healed tuberculosis)
- Persons with symptoms of infection in the lung, pleura, or airways, including larynx
- HIV–infected persons with any respiratory symptoms or signs, regardless of chest radiograph findings
- Persons suspected of having pulmonary tuberculosis disease for whom bronchoscopy is planned

Specimen collection for microbiology testing. The proper testing of sputum includes at least three specimens examined by smear and culture. The preferred method is to collect early morning specimens on three consecutive days. Specimens should be obtained in an isolated, well-ventilated space or in a sputum collection booth. It is recommended that a trained health care worker provide coaching and direct supervision for at least the first collection. An explanation about what type of specimen is acceptable (sputum) and that saliva and mucus from the nose or throat are not proper specimens should be given to the patient. Detailed coaching and supervision of the patient will expedite the testing process because unsupervised patients are not usually successful in providing an adequate specimen.

Some patients are unable to produce sputum by merely coughing. In these cases, the sputum specimen may be obtained by inducing a productive cough through the use of warm aerosol hypertonic saline. If this is not effective, a bronchoscopy may be performed. Bronchial washings, brushings, and biopsy specimens can be obtained through this procedure, and these specimens tested. In addition, gastric aspiration can be used to obtain specimens of swallowed sputum. This method is less invasive than a bronchoscopy and is an easier way to obtain specimens from infants and some young children when they cannot produce coughed sputum.

All of these procedures can produce an aerosol that is potentially contagious. Therefore, precautionary measures must be taken to reduce the risk to health care workers, and other patients should be removed from the area while specimens are being collected.

Although the most common specimen is sputum, tuberculosis infection can travel to many sites in the body. Other specimens can include cerebrospinal fluid, pleural fluid, pus, biopsy specimens from any anatomical site, and urine when extrapulmonary tuberculosis disease is suspected. Transport media is commonly used for tissue specimens, and all specimens should be delivered to the laboratory as soon as possible.

Infection Control for the Health Care Worker

It is essential that proper protection be provided for health care workers or others who are involved in specimen collection, transport, processing, and testing. If bronchoscopy or sputum induction procedures are used, there must be rooms dedicated to the procedure; the procedure needs to be scheduled when a minimum of health care workers are in attendance and when no other patients are present. Both procedures should be performed in a room that meets the requirements for an airborne infection isolation (AII) room, which includes negative airflow. Staff present during the procedure on a patient with suspected or confirmed tuberculosis need to wear an appropriate respirator during the procedure.

All sputum specimens or other specimens from known or suspected sites of tuberculosis infection need to be secured to protect whoever transports the specimen.

When the specimen reaches the laboratory, it should be handled with gloves. The laboratory staff who handles the specimens and performs testing should do so in a certified Class I or II biosafety cabinet, and should use Biosafety Level 3 practices, procedures, and containment equipment if any procedures are used that produce aerosols. For more on infection control, *see* Chapter 3.

Specimen Testing

The laboratory should perform an initial microscopic examination of stained smears for AFB. Fluorochrome staining is the preferred staining method because it is faster than the older, traditional methods. It is a quick procedure, but gives only a presumptive diagnosis of tuberculosis because identified AFB could be mycobacteria other than *M. tuberculosis*. In addition, many patients with tuberculosis disease have negative AFB smears.

Cultures should be performed on all specimens regardless of the results of the AFB smear. Positive cultures for *M. tuberculosis* confirm the diagnosis of tuberculosis disease. However, even with a negative culture, a diagnosis of tuberculosis can be made on the basis of clinical signs and symptoms.

After the mycobacteria have been grown in a culture, the species can be identified using nucleic acid probes. Nucleic acid amplification tests can be used to facilitate rapid detection of the microorganisms.

For all patients, the initial *M. tuberculosis* isolates need to be tested for drug resistance. It is of the utmost importance that drug resistance be identified as early as possible to ensure appropriate treatment.

It is up to the primary health care provider to promptly report all suspected or confirmed cases of tuberculosis to the appropriate health department as quickly as possible, as well as to report susceptibility results as they become available.

Isolation of Patients

During the time a patient is suspected of having infectious tuberculosis or is confirmed as having tuberculosis and is beginning treatment, environmental controls need to provide protection against the patient infecting other patients, staff members, and visitors. These controls include local exhaust ventilation, general ventilation, high-efficiency particulate air (HEPA) filtration, and ultraviolet germicidal irradiation (UVGI). The purpose of these controls, described in detail in Chapter 3, is to help prevent the spread and to reduce the concentration of airborne infectious droplet nuclei.

To separate patients who probably have infectious tuberculosis from others, health care facilities use AII rooms. Formerly known as negative-pressure rooms, AII rooms

---

Infectious Droplet Nuclei

Droplet nuclei produced by an infectious tuberculosis (TB) patient that can carry tubercle bacteria and be inhaled by others. Although usually produced from patients with pulmonary TB through coughing, aerosol-generating procedures can also generate infectious droplet nuclei.

---

are single-occupancy patient care rooms with specialized environmental controls to minimize the transmission of infectious agents from person to person. AII rooms should provide negative pressure in the room. This means that air does not flow from the room into other areas of the facility; rather, air from the room is ventilated directly to the outdoors or is recirculated through an HEPA filter. Although a properly maintained AII room will protect others in the facility, it does not protect those health care workers who come into close contact with the patient. Those health care workers should still take appropriate respiratory precautions, such as wearing a respirator. (*See* Chapter 3 for more information on respiratory protection controls.) If an organization does not have an appropriate space to isolate a patient, it should transfer the patient to a health care facility with appropriate space.

A patient who has drug-susceptible tuberculosis and has had a significant clinical and bacteriological response to a standard multidrug antituberculosis therapy is probably no longer infectious. These signs would probably be a reduction in cough, resolution of fever, and progressively decreasing quantity of AFB on the smear result. Because culture and susceptibility results usually take some time to become available, all patients with suspected tuberculosis should remain under airborne precautions while they are hospitalized until the following occurs:

- The patient has three negative AFB sputum smears, each of which should be collected in 8- to 24-hour intervals, and at least one of which should be an early morning specimen.
- The patient has received standard multidrug treatment for a minimum of two weeks and has demonstrated clinical improvement.

A hospitalized patient who is deemed medically stable can be discharged from the hospital before converting the positive AFB sputum smear to negative if the following criteria are met:

- A specific discharge plan is defined for follow-up care with the local tuberculosis control program.
- The patient has begun a standard multidrug antituberculosis treatment, and the process of directly observed therapy (DOT) has been arranged.
- No infants or children younger than 4 years old or persons with immunocompromising conditions are present in the household.
- All immunocompetent household members have been previously exposed to the patient.
- The patient is willing to abstain from travel outside the home except for health care–associated visits until he or she has negative sputum smear results.

Treatment

Treatment for Patients with LTBI

Treatment for LTBI substantially reduces the risk that infection with *M. tuberculosis* will progress to active tuberculosis disease. Therefore, it is of the utmost importance in the fight to control and eliminate tuberculosis disease to identify and treat individuals with LTBI. The CDC, the World Health Organization (WHO), and other interested professional groups have identified groups of people who are at a higher risk of developing tuberculosis disease after being infected and who would therefore be at a high priority for treatment. These individuals should be given treatment, and ongoing efforts should be made to assure they have completed the course of treatment.

It is recommended that the following individuals receive treatment if the induration from a TST is equal to or greater than 5 mm, regardless of age:
- Persons infected with HIV
- Persons who have had recent contact with someone with tuberculosis disease
- Individuals with fibrotic changes in a chest radiograph consistent with previous tuberculosis disease
- Organ transplant recipients
- Other immunosuppressed individuals (for example, those being medicated with at least 15 mg/day of prednisone for a month or more)

The following groups should be considered for treatment if the TST result is equal to or greater than 10 mm, or if the blood assay for *M. tuberculosis* (BAMT) is positive for the following:
- Those with TST or BAMT conversions
- Individuals born or who have lived in developing countries or countries with a high incidence of tuberculosis disease
- Persons who inject illicit drugs
- Residents and employees in congregate settings that are at high risk, such as correctional facilities, long term care facilities (hospices and skilled nursing facilities), hospitals and other health care facilities, residential settings for persons with HIV/AIDS or other immunosuppressed conditions, and homeless shelters
- Personnel from mycobacteriology laboratories
- Individuals with any of the following conditions or other immunocompromising conditions that would put them at high risk for tuberculosis disease:
  - Silicosis
  - Diabetes mellitus

- Chronic renal failure
- Hematologic disorders such as leukemias and lymphomas
- Other specific malignancies, such as carcinoma of the head, neck, or lung
- Unexplained weight loss of 10% or more of the person's ideal body weight
- Gastrectomy
- Jejunoileal bypass
- Those living in areas with a high incidence of tuberculosis disease
- Children under the age of 4 years
- Infants, children, and adolescents exposed to adults at high risk for developing tuberculosis disease

Persons with no known risk factors can be considered for treatment if their TST induration is equal to or greater than 15 mm.

Before beginning treatment for LTBI, the clinician needs to rule out tuberculosis disease using a medical history, medical examination, chest radiography, and, when indicated, bacteriologic studies. In addition, it is important to ensure that the patient has not had adverse reactions with previous isoniazid (INH) treatment. Patients with a previous history of liver injury or excessive alcohol consumption might not be good candidates for treatment of LTBI. Active hepatitis and end-stage liver disease are relative contraindications to the use of INH. If a decision is made to treat such patients, baseline and follow-up testing of serum aminotransaminases should be used to monitor the patient.

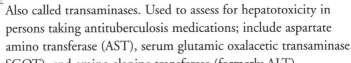

Aminotransaminases
Also called transaminases. Used to assess for hepatotoxicity in persons taking antituberculosis medications; include aspartate amino transferase (AST), serum glutamic oxalacetic transaminase (formerly SGOT), and amino alanine transferase (formerly ALT).

Persons who are in contact with patients with drug-susceptible tuberculosis disease and who previously had a negative TST or BAMT result and subsequently had a positive TST or BAMT result of equal to or greater than 5 mm should be evaluated for treatment of LTBI. The majority of people who are infected with *M. tuberculosis* will have a positive TST result within 6 weeks of exposure. Therefore, contacts with negative TST or BAMT results should be retested 8 to 10 weeks after the end of exposure to a patient with suspected or confirmed tuberculosis disease.

Some close contacts of persons with tuberculosis disease also need to be evaluated for treatment of LTBI after tuberculosis disease has been ruled out. These persons include the following:
• Children under the age of 4 years
• Immunosuppressed persons
• Others who may develop tuberculosis disease quickly after infection

Close contacts who have a negative reaction to an initial TST need to be retested 10 to 12 weeks after they were last exposed to tuberculosis. Meanwhile, treatment should begin. Treatment may then be discontinued if the test is again negative. However, if an individual is known to have or suspected of having HIV infection, he or she should be given LTBI treatment regardless of the test result. This can also apply to other immunocompromised people.

Infants and young children with LTBI are by their very age determined to have been infected recently and are at risk of the infection progressing to tuberculosis disease. They are also more likely to develop life-threatening forms of tuberculosis. Therefore, close contacts in this age group need to receive treatment even if test results are negative because they may be anergic. Treatment of LTBI can be discontinued if all the following conditions are met:
• The infant is at least 6 months old
• The second test given 10 to 12 weeks after the last exposure to infectious tuberculosis disease is also negative

Several regimens are available for treating LTBI, and it is suggested that clinicians discuss options with their patients. For patients who are at high risk for tuberculosis disease and who may be noncompliant with taking medication or are on intermittent dosing regimen, DOT should be considered.

Antibiotics generally used for treating LTBI include the following:
• Isoniazid (INH)
• Rifampin (RIF)
• Pyrazinamide (PZA)

Other antibiotics that may be used when these present a problem or there is resistance include the following:
• Rifambutin

- A Quinolone (levofloxacin, ofloxacin, or ciprofloxacin)
- Ethambutol

Treatment for Patients with Tuberculosis Disease

Suspected or confirmed tuberculosis cases are required to be reported to the local or state health department. Case management for tuberculosis disease needs to be coordinated with officials of the relevant health department. Regimens for treatment of tuberculosis disease must contain multiple drugs to which the organism is susceptible. Treatment using multiple drugs is based on two principles: preventing acquired drug resistance and enhancing efficacy. Treatment of tuberculosis disease with a single drug can lead to the development of mycobacterial resistance to that drug.

For the majority of patients, the preferred regimen consists of an initial two-month treatment of four drugs (INH, RIF, PZA, and ethambutol) and a four-month continuation phase of INH and RIF. The minimum total treatment time is, therefore, six months. Based on supporting drug susceptibility testing, ethambutol may be discontinued for some patients. The criteria for completing therapy are based on the number of doses taken within the maximal period, and not simply the six-month time frame. Patients with cavitary pulmonary tuberculosis disease and positive sputum culture results at the end of two months of therapy need to receive a longer continuation phase (seven months) because of the significantly higher chances of relapse.

For patients with HIV who are on antiretroviral therapy, it is best to have treatment provided by or in consultation with someone who is an expert in the management of both HIV and tuberculosis. The tuberculosis treatment regimen might need to be altered for these patients; if the patient has CD4 cell counts of less than 100 cells/cubic millimeter, the patient should not be treated with intermittent regimens of once or twice a week. These patients should receive daily treatment during the intensive phase by DOT and daily or three times a week treatment by DOT during the continuation phase.

The most important determinant of successful outcomes of treatment is careful adherence to the drug regimen. Therefore, with all cases, care should be taken to ensure that the regimen is followed by using measures that enable and foster adherence. Figure 2-1, page 57, shows U.S. rates of treatment completion.

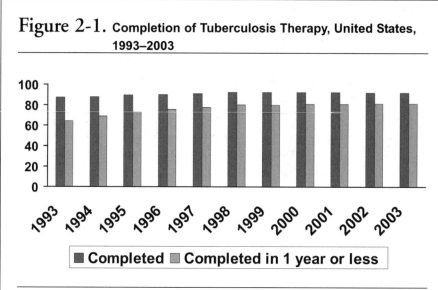

Figure 2-1. Completion of Tuberculosis Therapy, United States, 1993–2003

■ Completed ■ Completed in 1 year or less

Source: Centers for Disease Control and Prevention: *2005 Surveillance Slides: Completion of TB Therapy: United States, 1993–2003.* http://www.cdc.gov/tb/pubs/slidesets/surv/surv2005/Slides/surv26.htm (accessed Oct. 3, 2007).

Treatment interruptions are problematic as well. One study of patients in 1998 and 1999 found that 6% of patients had treatment interruptions; the median number of months to treatment interruption was four. The biggest factors in these interruptions, the study found, were homelessness and a lack of awareness of the severity of tuberculosis.[8] Sidebar 2-2, page 58, has more information about the association between tuberculosis and homelessness.

Incomplete or inadequate treatment can lead to the following:
• Relapse of the patient
• Continued transmission
• Development of drug resistance

There are important steps that need to be taken to obtain maximum benefit from treatment. These include patient education, case management, and DOT.

All patients or their caregiver(s) need to receive education on the following:
• Tuberculosis disease

Sidebar 2-2.
Tuberculosis and Homelessness

It's not surprising that homeless people are particularly at risk for contracting tuberculosis and for interrupting treatment. Lack of adequate health care prevents latent infections from being discovered before they become tuberculosis disease, and when the disease is diagnosed, it is difficult for health care facilities to follow up with patients to ensure that they continue all necessary treatment. Health care facilities that tend to encounter homeless patients should make particular efforts to diagnose and treat these individuals completely and appropriately.

A 2005 CDC study found that homeless people also tend to have other risk factors that can affect tuberculosis diagnosis and treatment. For example, homeless people have a higher rate of substance abuse than nonhomeless people, and 34% have HIV coinfection. In addition, although homeless tuberculosis patients were not more likely to have a drug-resistant strain of the disease, they were more likely to be infectious than nonhomeless patients.

The study also found that correctional facilities play a large role in diagnosing these patients. Many of the homeless tuberculosis cases are discovered in local jails: At the time of tuberculosis diagnosis, 9% of homeless tuberculosis patients were incarcerated.

Source: Haddad M.B., et al.: Tuberculosis and homelessness in the United States, 1994–2003. *JAMA* 293:2762–2766, Jun. 8, 2005.

- The medication (dosing, possible adverse effects, and how important it is to take the medication according to instructions); verbal and written instructions should be given.

For more on patient and health care worker education, *see* Chapter 4.

Case management requires a person to be assigned responsibility for the patient, some form of regular review of the case, and a process to correct or lessen problems with compliance.

DOT is a process that has resulted in significant improvements in the compliance rates of persons on tuberculosis treatment regimens. It requires that a health care worker or other designated individual observe the patient swallow each dose of tuberculosis medication. This requires intensive oversight, but is so successful that it is a vital part of the WHO's *The Global Plan to Stop TB 2006–2015*. DOT should be considered for all tuberculosis patients, but it requires a great deal of coordination to be successful. The use of this approach has a significant effect on decreasing drug resistance.

It is important that DOT be used where it is convenient for the patient. In some settings, such as nursing homes or other settings where the patient may be institutionalized, it is far easier to implement. However, home health workers or designated family or community members may be used for the purpose. When a patient is unable or unwilling to consistently meet the medication regimen requirements, the health department should be notified. The health department should be able to assist the responsible clinician in providing services to help the patient to comply with the therapy regimen. When lack of compliance cannot be modified, even with strong encouragement and health department intervention, enforced quarantine is sometimes necessary.

Diagnosing and Treating Patients with Special Circumstances

Patients with HIV/AIDS

A review of data from the WHO, the Joint United Nations Programme on HIV/Acquired Immunodeficiency Syndrome, the U.S. Census Bureau, and the CDC indicates that tuberculosis is the cause of death for 11% of all AIDS patients.[9] In addition, 7% to 12% of all new tuberculosis cases worldwide in adults 15 to 49 are attributable to HIV infection; in the United States, that proportion is 26%—one of the highest rates for industrialized nations. The percentage and absolute number of patients with tuberculosis disease who are infected with HIV-1 (the most common form of the virus) are declining in the United States because of improved infection control practices and better diagnosis and treatment of both HIV-1 infection and tuberculosis. With increased voluntary counseling and testing and the increasing use of treatment for LTBI, tuberculosis disease will probably continue to decrease among HIV-1–infected persons in the United States and Western Europe.[10] But this can happen only with continued expertise and vigilance. It takes specialized expertise to diagnose and treat patients with coinfection of HIV/AIDS and tuberculosis.

The degree of immunodeficiency greatly influences the presentation of the disease. HIV-1–related tuberculosis appears like tuberculosis among persons not infected with HIV. The majority of patients have disease limited to the lungs, and common chest radiographic manifestations include upper lobe fibronodular infiltrates with or without cavitation. However, extrapulmonary tuberculosis disease is more common in patients with HIV-1 than in non–HIV infected persons. When extrapulmonary disease occurs in HIV-1–infected persons, clinical manifestations are not substantially different from those described in patients not infected with HIV.

As a person's degree of immunodeficiency increases, extrapulmonary tuberculosis, with or without pulmonary involvement, becomes more common. Among severely immunocompromised patients, tuberculosis can be a severe systemic disease with high fevers, rapid progression, and sepsis syndrome. The chest radiographic findings of tuberculosis disease in advanced AIDS are markedly different compared with those among patients with less severe HIV-1 infection; lower lobe, middle lobe, and miliary infiltrates are common, and cavitation is less common. Patients with HIV-1 infection and pulmonary tuberculosis can have sputum smears and culture results positive for AFB or *M. tuberculosis,* respectively, even with a normal chest radiograph.

To make a diagnosis of tuberculosis with HIV–infected individuals, the following should be kept in mind:
- Sputum samples with these patients are often negative by direct smear microscopy.
- Among patients with more severe immunodeficiency, sputum smear and culture examinations become somewhat less sensitive than in patents with relatively intact immune systems, and TST has limited diagnostic value because it is often negative.
- Sputum samples for smear and culture need to be obtained from patients with pulmonary symptoms, cervical adenopathy, or chest radiographic abnormalities.
- The evaluation of suspected tuberculosis in these patients should always include a chest radiograph.
- For patients with signs of extrapulmonary tuberculosis, needle aspiration of skin lesions, nodes, or fluids (pleural, pericardial) can provide rapid diagnosis, culture, and susceptibility testing; in cases in which fine-needle aspirates are negative, tissue biopsies can be helpful.
- When there are signs of disseminated disease, blood cultures might allow for a definitive diagnosis. Mycobacterial blood cultures are more sensitive for diagnosis of tuberculosis in severely immunodeficient patients.

- For patients with relatively intact immune function, the results of sputum smear and culture examinations are similar to that of adults not infected with HIV, with positive smear results being more common among patients with cavitary pulmonary involvement.
- Any specimen that is smear positive in HIV/AIDS patients should be treated as positive for tuberculosis until species identification can be made because of the virulence of *M. tuberculosis* in this patient population.
- Drug susceptibility testing and adjustment of the treatment regimen based on the results are critical to the successful treatment of tuberculosis and to prevention of transmission of drug-resistant *M. tuberculosis* in the community. Therefore, the following testing should be done:
  a. For all specimens, testing for susceptibility to first-line agents (INH, RIF, and ethambutol) should be performed.
  b. PZA susceptibility testing should be performed if there is a sufficiently high rate of PZA resistance in the community.
  c. Only reference laboratories should perform second-line drug susceptibility testing.
  d. Second-line drug susceptibility testing should be limited to specimens from patients who meet at least one of the following criteria:
     – Have had previous therapy
     – Are contacts of patients with drug-resistant tuberculosis disease
     – Have demonstrated resistance to RIF or to other first-line drugs
     – Have positive cultures after at least three months of treatment

Elderly Patients in Long Term Care Facilities

Because the elderly often have health concerns that make them more susceptible to infection, they are at higher risk for tuberculosis than the general population. Older people who live in nursing homes are particularly vulnerable, not only because of reactivation from prior infection, but because they may also become infected from being in close contact with another resident who is infectious. Geriatric care providers must be aware of this increased risk and have a tuberculosis infection control plan in place to prevent and control tuberculosis in long term care facilities.

Most cases of tuberculosis disease for geriatric patients are found in those who live in communities, such as long term care facilities. CDC guidelines recommend a two-step TST for all new residents and employees as soon as their residency or employment begins unless they have documentation of a previous positive reaction. It is important to remember that in this population there can be both false positives (from exposure to atypical mycobacteria in the environment) and false negatives (because of the inability to produce an adequate immune response required to demonstrate a positive result). In addition, previous vaccination with BCG can cause false positives. However, the effect of vaccination with BCG on reactivity to TST or protection from the disease itself has not been well described in older adults. Consequently, there should be a strong suspicion of LTBI in an older resident with a positive TST result, even if there has been a history of BCG vaccination. This is particularly true when the patient has come from an area where tuberculosis is endemic. False negative results on the TST are found in patients with overwhelming tuberculosis disease (miliary tuberculosis), with HIV infection, receiving immunosuppressive therapy, and with malnutrition and the elderly. Therefore, in elderly patients, a negative TST result should not lead the clinician to rule out tuberculosis disease.

Each person whose TST or BAMT converts to positive should have a chest radiograph; if the radiograph is negative for tuberculosis, the individual should be treated preventively. If the source of infection is not known and/or if additional conversions occur, periodic retesting of residents and a careful search for the source case should be continued.

Individuals with reactions greater than or equal to 10 mm and those with symptoms suggesting tuberculosis (for example, cough, anorexia, weight loss, fever), regardless of the size of the skin test reaction, should have a chest radiograph within 72 hours. Persons with abnormal chest radiographs and/or symptoms compatible with tuberculosis should also have sputum smear and culture examinations. In addition, sputum should be submitted for smear and culture for AFB for persons with a chronic cough, pneumonia, or bronchitis who do not respond promptly and completely to antibiotic treatment. At least three sputum specimens should be submitted. In the absence of spontaneous production of sputum, suction of laryngeal or pharyngeal mucus is satisfactory if sterile water is used in clearing the catheter. Usually, the early detection of tuberculosis by such means either prevents or greatly diminishes the spread of infection.

Staff members who are considered to have infectious tuberculosis should be relieved of responsibilities until the diagnosis is excluded or until they become noninfectious as a result of effective chemotherapy.[11]

It is typical of radiographs of old tuberculosis disease to include calcified granulomas, scars, fibrosis, or thickened apical pleura. Older patients with these manifestations are at increased risk of developing reactivation of the disease. A chest x-ray with these results in a setting of nonspecific signs and symptoms of disease can provide important information that reactivation has occurred. It is possible that classic findings on the radiographs, such as lung cavitation, may be reduced in elderly patients with the disease. It is recommended that tuberculosis disease be considered in elderly residents if symptoms and abnormalities on the radiograph strongly suggest the diagnosis or if the long term care resident fails to respond to therapy for more common causes of lower respiratory tract infection.

Children with Tuberculosis

Extrapulmonary and miliary tuberculosis is more common among younger children. In addition, younger children are more likely to progress more rapidly from infection to active disease than older children and adults; they also may have negative skin tests and fewer symptoms of disease, and, therefore, the diagnosis is easier to miss.

Congenital tuberculosis is rare but has been reported among children born to HIV–infected women with active tuberculosis. The mother might not have symptoms of tuberculosis disease, and subclinical maternal genital tuberculosis also can result in an infected neonate.

Children with tuberculosis disease are almost always infected by an adult in their daily environment,[12,13] and, because of the patients' youth, it can be assumed that the infection represents primary infection rather than the reactivation disease sometimes observed among adults. Identification and treatment of the source patient and evaluation of all exposed children is particularly important; all confirmed and suspected tuberculosis cases should be reported to state and local health departments, which will assist in contact evaluation. In addition, other exposed members of the household should be evaluated because other secondary tuberculosis cases and latent infections with *M. tuberculosis* often are found. Latent infections should be treated to prevent active cases.

Because it is difficult to isolate *M. tuberculosis* from a child with pulmonary tuberculosis, it is frequently necessary to rely on the results of drug susceptibility tests of the organisms isolated from the presumed source case to guide the choice of drugs for the child. In cases of suspected drug-resistant tuberculosis in a child or when a source-case isolate is not available, specimens for microbiological evaluation should be obtained via early morning gastric aspiration, bronchoalveolar lavage, or biopsy.

Because of the high risk of disseminated tuberculosis in infants and children younger than 4 years of age, treatment should be started as soon as the diagnosis of tuberculosis is suspected. In general, the regimens recommended for adults are also the regimens of choice for infants, children, and adolescents; however, ethambutol is not used routinely in children. In most cases of tuberculosis in children, there is less concern with the development of acquired drug resistance. Children and adolescents may develop tuberculosis with upper lobe infiltration, cavitation, and sputum production, in much the same way as adults. In such situations an initial phase of four drugs should be given until susceptibility is proven. When clinical or epidemiologic circumstances suggest an increased probability of INH resistance, ethambutol can be used safely at a dose of 15–20 mg/kg per day, even in children too young for routine eye testing.

Most studies of treatment in children have used six months of INH and RIF supplemented during the first two months with PZA. This three-drug combination has a success rate of greater than 95% and an adverse drug reaction rate of less than 2%. Most treatment studies of intermittent dosing in children have used daily drug administration for the first two weeks to two months. DOT should always be used in treating children.

In general, extrapulmonary tuberculosis in children can be treated with the same regimens as pulmonary disease. Exceptions are disseminated tuberculosis and tuberculous meningitis, for which there are inadequate data to support 6-month therapy; thus 9 to 12 months of treatment is recommended.

The optimal treatment of pulmonary tuberculosis in children and adolescents with HIV infection is unknown. The American Academy of Pediatrics recommends that initial therapy always include at least three drugs, and that the total duration of therapy be at least nine months, although there are no data to support this recommendation.[14,15]

Persons in Correctional Institutions

Compared with the general population, inmates of correctional facilities have higher tuberculosis rates due to a higher prevalence of HIV infection and substance abuse and lower socioeconomic status. The risk for transmission is increased because of close living conditions, poor ventilation, and overcrowding.

The following case study can demonstrate the problems inherent with this population, and with diagnosing and treating tuberculosis patients in general.

CASE STUDY 2-1. TUBERCULOSIS INFECTION IN CORRECTIONAL FACILITIES

In 2001 and 2002 a man with active tuberculosis disease was held for a total of 14 weeks in three jails, none of which had a tuberculosis infection-control plan (TBICP). He was ultimately sent to a Kansas state prison, where he answered affirmatively to six of seven questions about tuberculosis symptoms. However, he was not referred for a medical evaluation. The two-step TST given to all entering prisoners was read as 0 mm induration for both tests. The inmate was placed among the general prison population. He was not seen medically until four weeks later, when he was given a medical examination for the asthma that had been misdiagnosed during an earlier incarceration. At this time, he received a chest radiograph that showed a cavitary lesion of the right lower lobe. Even though he had tuberculosis symptoms and a positive radiograph, he was put back with the general prison population, and was scheduled for a CT scan to rule out neoplasia. After the CT scan two weeks later, the man was identified as a tuberculosis patient and placed in AII. The AII room was new and in working order. However, the recommended N95 respirator masks were not available; prison health care workers used surgical masks when in the room with the patient.

The contact investigation identified 318 of an estimated 800 possible contacts of the patient. Two contacts had a diagnosis of tuberculosis disease. Of the 318 contacts, 256 were tested, and 47 received a diagnosis of LTBI.

As a result of the investigation of this case, the Kansas Tuberculosis Control Program worked with prisons, jails, and local health departments to provide guidelines for developing or improving TBICPs and to provide tuberculosis education and baseline TSTs for all correctional employees. This guidance has improved communication among all agencies to coordinate the return to the community of inmates receiving tuberculosis medications.[16]

The CDC recommendations for a TBICP in a correctional facility are discussed in the following sections.

Goal of TBICP in Correctional Facilities
- Prevent disease transmission by enabling early identification and prompt initiation of treatment of tuberculosis disease.

Screen Inmates
- Identify inmates with tuberculosis disease and LTBI promptly.
- Follow guidelines of the Advisory Council for the Elimination of Tuberculosis for screening based on correctional facility type.
- Report cases of suspected or confirmed tuberculosis disease to the health department.

Isolate Persons with Suspected or Confirmed Tuberculosis Disease
- Use an AII room within the facility or transfer the patient to a local hospital where an AII room is available.
- Instruct persons who enter the AII room to wear N95 respirators.
- Implement a thorough contact investigation promptly.

Treat Persons with Tuberculosis Disease and LTBI
- Provide appropriate diagnostic, treatment, and laboratory services.
- Follow American Thoracic Society treatment guidelines.
- Perform DOT with all tuberculosis medications.
- Follow up with inmates released before completing treatment.

Assess Tuberculosis Prevention Activities
- Monitor and evaluate screening and containment efforts.
- Collect and analyze data to monitor whether these activities are being implemented successfully.

Implement and Maintain Engineering Controls
- Ensure that all engineering controls are properly installed and maintained.
- Consider supplementing ventilation systems in temporary holding and communal areas with HEPA filtration and UVGI.

Employee Protection Program
- Obtain medical history, provide physical examinations, and perform TST for all new employees at the time of hiring.
- Implement a formal respiratory protection program, including employee education and fit testing for respirator use.

Homeless Populations

In 2003, as the incidence of tuberculosis cases in the United States declined, 6.3% of the reported cases were among homeless persons.[17] A review of a reported case in New York City exemplifies the inherent problems with diagnosing and treating the homeless.[18] Between January and July 2003, four tuberculosis cases were reported by the Orange County Health Department, New York, among residents of a homeless shelter for men. When the New York State Department of Health communicated the occurrences of these four cases to the New York City Department of Health and Mental Hygiene, the latter department had identified four additional tuberculosis cases among residents of the same shelter for the same time interval. At this point, a joint investigation of the cluster was undertaken. The following are three factors that led to a decision to conduct an intensive active case investigation:

1. Identification of two long term care residents with AFB sputum smear with positive pulmonary tuberculosis in August 2003
2. Newly identified HIV coinfections in four of the tuberculosis patients
3. Suspicion of recent tuberculosis transmission in the shelter

The patients were screened using tuberculosis symptom surveys, chest radiographs, and TSTs. Of the 1,038 residents, 958 were registered for the screening and interviewed for tuberculosis symptoms and HIV risk factors. Among the residents screened, 927 (97%) had a chest radiograph and 593 (62%) had TSTs given, with 583 having TSTs read. Of these 583 TSTs read, 223 were positive (using the criteria of an induration equal to or greater than 5 mm). Treatment with INH was provided at the shelter for 161 of the 225 residents for whom LTBI treatment using DOT was recommended. Fast-food coupons were provided to encourage adherence to completing the therapy.

From 2000 to 2003, 29 tuberculosis cases were identified among residents of this facility. Of those for which genotyping was available, 11 cases shared the same *M. tuberculosis* genotype. The earliest case identified with this strain was a patient who had culture-confirmed pulmonary tuberculosis diagnosed on three occasions. The first two occasions were in 1996 and 2000 when the patient did not complete treatment before being lost to follow-up, and the third was in April 2001, six months after the patient had entered the shelter with his tuberculosis status unknown to shelter staff. One patient outside the shelter who was diagnosed with the same strain had worked with the probable source patient in 2000.

Of the 297 shelter workers, 228 were assessed for tuberculosis. Of these, 16 (7%) showed newly positive TST results. Tuberculosis disease was not identified among the workers.

The following are some of the problems noted after this investigation and after other outbreaks:

- There is rapid progression of the disease in shelters for persons coinfected with HIV.
- Notification of cases to three different local health departments and incomplete sharing of information between these departments masked the extent of tuberculosis disease and transmission in this population until the departments began communicating with each other.
- Some cases were not initially associated with the shelter because of homelessness and varying methods of recording addresses.
- Failure of persons in this population to complete treatment increase the ability of the disease to spread; in this outbreak, 11 tuberculosis cases could have been prevented if the index patient with the shelter-associated strain had completed his treatment when the tuberculosis was diagnosed in 1996 or in 2000.

Because tuberculosis is a major problem among homeless persons, the CDC's Advisory Council for the Elimination of Tuberculosis developed recommendations to assist all those who minister to this population and the affected persons themselves prevent and control tuberculosis.

The exact number of people considered homeless is not known at any given time, and in fact, estimates are widely varied. Even the incidence of active tuberculosis and of LTBI among the homeless is unknown. However, based on screening at specific clinics and shelters, the rate of active tuberculosis disease has a range from 1.6% to 6.8%; the rate of LTBI has a range from 18% to 51%. Although shelters for the homeless are very important for the survival of these individuals, they also provide a common space where tuberculosis can be transmitted more readily than in a home, particularly in the winter when shelters are more likely to be crowded and not adequately ventilated.

The following are recommendations for prevention and control of tuberculosis among homeless persons made by the Advisory Council for the Elimination of Tuberculosis, listed in the order of priority[19]:

1. The highest priority should be given to the following:

    a. Detection, evaluation, and reporting of homeless persons who have current symptoms of active tuberculosis

    b. Completion of an appropriate course of treatment by those diagnosed with active tuberculosis

2. The second priority should be screening and preventive therapy for homeless persons who have, or are suspected of having, HIV infection.

3. The third priority should be the examination and appropriate treatment of persons with recent tuberculosis that has been inadequately treated.

4. The fourth priority should be screening and appropriate treatment of persons exposed to an infectious (sputum-positive) case of tuberculosis. Because contacts are difficult to define in a shelter population, it is usually necessary to screen all residents of a shelter when an infectious case is identified.

5. The fifth priority should be screening and preventive therapy for homeless persons with known medical conditions that increase the risk of tuberculosis (for example, diabetes mellitus).

Priorities for preventive therapy among tuberculosis-infected persons are as follows:
1. Those with HIV infection
2. Recent contacts of persons with infectious tuberculosis
3. Those with recent skin test conversions or BAMT conversions
4. Those with tuberculosis disease who have been inadequately treated
5. Persons with negative sputum cultures and stable fibrotic lesions on chest radiographs consistent with inactive tuberculosis
6. Individuals with medical conditions that increase the risk of tuberculosis

Foreign-Born Populations

What the statistics show us about this population includes the following:

- Compared with U.S.-born patients, a higher percentage of non–U.S.-born patients have extrapulmonary tuberculosis only.
- Drug-resistance rates are higher among non–U.S.-born populations than among the U.S. born.
- The outcome of tuberculosis treatment is slightly better for non–U.S.-born patients than for U.S.-born patients.
- In the United States, HIV has not played a major role in tuberculosis cases among non–U.S.-born persons in most areas. The only exception is persons from Haiti. Recent studies conducted in southern Florida indicated that half of the Haitians infected with tuberculosis among those age 25–44 were also HIV positive.

The above statistics are taken from CDC's *Morbidity and Mortality Weekly Report: Recommendations and Reports* of September 18, 1998, entitled "Recommendations for Prevention and Control of Tuberculosis Among Foreign-Born Persons: Report of the Working Group on Tuberculosis Among Foreign-Born Persons." This report details recommendations for the CDC, as well as state and local public health departments. It highlights the need for health care organizations to maintain communication with their public health departments. More information regarding tuberculosis risks among non–U.S.-born patients can be found in Chapter 1.

Foreign-born persons encounter cultural and structural barriers in being able and willing to access the health system in the United States. Some of these challenges include the following:
- Language and other communication difficulties
- Cultural barriers, including the stigma of tuberculosis in their own country
- Not knowing how to access the health system in this country
- Being uninsured and unable to afford health care
- For undocumented persons, fear of being discovered and deported

Any of these issues can cause the individual to delay seeking health care. This, in turn expands the numbers and intensities of contacts. It also means that the disease will have progressed further and require more expensive care when a diagnosis is made.

The problems linked to noncompletion of treatment can be caused by the same issues that delay or impede these persons from seeking treatment and include the following:
- Nonadherence to the treatment regimen
- Inadequate tracking systems
- Information gaps
- Drug resistance

The problems with tracking and communication systems relate in great part to the mobility of many non–U.S.-born individuals, such as migrant and seasonal farm workers who move among states and countries while under treatment. In these cases, health departments are unable to track and refer these patients to assure that treatment is completed. Also, others return to their country of origin before completion of treatment, with no follow-up care. Essentially no communication exists between tuberculosis controllers in the United States and their counterparts in foreign countries, with the exception of the U.S.-Mexico border region where lines of communication are being established.

There are special considerations for non–U.S.-born patients who were treated in their home countries. These include the following[20]:

- U.S. caregivers may not have access to the medical records of patients who were previously treated in another country.
- If the records are available, the medical information is likely to be in an unfamiliar language or format.
- National tuberculosis control program reports from countries that are sources of large numbers of tuberculosis cases among the foreign born often lack reliable data regarding rates of relapse, drug resistance, and completion of therapy.
- Because resources for tuberculosis control programs are severely limited in many foreign countries, persons treated for tuberculosis in these countries might receive inadequate or incomplete treatment. Thus, these individuals are at greater risk for disease recurrence with drug-resistant strains, which complicates and lengthens the course of treatment. Some persons with multiple resistant strains are chronically ill and persistently infectious. Although the total number of these patients with treatment-resistant tuberculosis is small, the cost associated with their medical care is many times that of patients with drug-susceptible disease. Treating these patients can severely strain local health department resources, particularly because non–U.S.-born populations are disproportionately underinsured or uninsured.

These issues make it imperative that tuberculosis in the non–U.S.-born population be dealt with aggressively, which the CDC is addressing, along with state and local departments of health. However, it is also important that health care professionals be aware of tuberculosis as a possible diagnosis when treating this group of patients (*see* Chapter 5).

Persons with Multidrug-Resistant Tuberculosis

Contacts who are considered likely to be newly infected and who have had exposure to a person with infectious multidrug-resistant tuberculosis (MDR-TB) need to be evaluated to assess the likelihood of infection with a multidrug-resistant strain of *M. tuberculosis*. The factors that should be addressed during the assessment are listed below.

Infectiousness of the Source Case

Tuberculosis patients who cough and have AFB smear–positive sputum are substantially more infectious than those who do not cough and have AFB smear–negative sputum. Evidence of TST conversions among contacts of the tuberculosis case is another measure of infectivity.

Closeness and Intensity of the MDR-TB Exposure

Any person who shared the air space with an MDR-TB patient for a relatively prolonged time (for example, household member, hospital roommate) is at higher risk for infection than those who had brief exposure to an MDR-TB patient, such as a one-time hospital visitor. Exposure of any length in a small, enclosed, poorly ventilated area is more likely to result in transmission than exposure in a large, well-ventilated space. Exposure during cough-inducing procedures (for example, bronchoscopy, endotracheal intubation, sputum induction, administration of aerosol therapy), which may greatly enhance tuberculosis transmission, is also more likely to result in infection.

Bronchoscopy

A procedure for examining the lower respiratory tract in which the end of the endoscopic instrument is inserted through the mouth or nose (or tracheostomy) and into the respiratory tree. Bronchoscopy can be used to obtain diagnostic specimens. Bronchoscopy also creates a high risk for *M. tuberculosis* transmission to health care workers if it is performed on an untreated patient who has tuberculosis disease (even if the patient has negative AFB smear results) because it is a cough-inducing procedure.

Contact History

Persons exposed to several sources of *M. tuberculosis,* including infectious tuberculosis patients with drug-susceptible *M. tuberculosis,* are less likely to have been infected with a multidrug-resistant strain than are those whose only known exposure to tuberculosis was to an infectious MDR-TB case.

Preventive Therapy Considerations for Persons Likely to Be Infected with MDR-TB

Before any preventive therapy regimen is initiated, the clinician needs to exclude the diagnosis of active tuberculosis disease. Patients on preventive therapy should be monitored carefully for adverse reactions to the medications, evidence of active tuberculosis, and adherence to therapy. They should also be educated about symptoms of tuberculosis and the need for immediate medical evaluation if symptoms do occur. As much as possible, alternative multidrug preventive therapy regimens should be selected, administered, and evaluated in a consistent and systematic way. All patients receiving one of these regimens should be on DOT.

Clinicians who are not familiar with the management of patients with MDR-TB or patients infected with multidrug-resistant organisms should seek expert consultation.

Considerations in Evaluating *M. tuberculosis* Isolates for Drug Susceptibility

Drug susceptibility test results of the *M. tuberculosis* isolate of the presumed source case should be considered in the selection of the drugs to be included in the preventive therapy regimen. The proportion method is commonly used for determining drug susceptibility of *M. tuberculosis* isolates. The results of this method of testing are reported to the clinician as the percentage of the total bacterial population resistant to a given drug, which is defined by the amount of growth on a drug-containing medium as compared with growth on a drug-free control medium. When greater than or equal to 1% of the bacillary population becomes resistant to the critical concentration of a drug, the *M. tuberculosis* isolate is considered resistant to that drug. The critical concentration of a drug is the concentration that inhibits the growth of most cells in wild strains of *M. tuberculosis.* One critical concentration is used for the susceptibility testing of most drugs; INH susceptibility testing is usually done by using two different drug concentrations (0.2 µg/mL and 1.0 µg/mL).[21]

References

1. Glassroth J.: Tuberculosis 2004: Challenges and opportunities. *Trans Am Clin Climatol Assoc* 116:293–309, 2005.

2. Centers for Disease Control and Prevention: Guidelines for preventing the transmission of *Mycobacterium tuberculosis* in health-care settings, 2005. *MMWR Recomm Rep* 54:1–147, Dec. 30, 2005.

3. Centers for Disease Control and Prevention (CDC): *Core Curriculum on Tuberculosis: What the Clinician Should Know,* 4th ed. Atlanta: CDC, 2000.

4. Williams V.G.: Tuberculosis: Clinical features, diagnosis and management. *Nurs Stand* 20(22):49–53, 2006.

5. Sokolove P., Rossman L., Cohen S.: The emergency department presentation of patients with active pulmonary tuberculosis. *Acad Emerg Med* 7:1056–1060, 2000.

6. Kanyana A.M., Gliddent D.V., Chambers H.F.: Identifying pulmonary tuberculosis in patients with negative sputum smear results. *Chest* 120:349–355, Aug. 2001.

7. Rozovsky-Weinberger J., et al.: Delays in suspicion and isolation among hospitalized persons with pulmonary tuberculosis at public and private U.S. hospitals during 1996 to 1999. *Chest* 127:205–212, 2005.

8. Driver C.R., et al.: Factors associated with tuberculosis treatment interruption in New York City. *J Public Health Manag Pract* 11:361–368, 2005.

9. Corbett E.L.: The growing burden of tuberculosis: Global trends and interactions with the HIV epidemic. *Arch Intern Med* 163:1009–1021, May 12, 2003.

10. Benson C.A., et al.: Treating opportunistic infections among HIV-infected adults and adolescents. *MMWR Recomm Rep* 53:1–112, Dec. 17, 2004.

11. Centers for Disease Control and Prevention: Prevention and control of tuberculosis in facilities providing long-term care to the elderly: Recommendations of the Advisory Committee for Elimination of Tuberculosis. *MMWR Recomm Rep* 39:7–20, Jul. 13, 1990.

12. Munoz F.: Tuberculosis among adult visitors of children with suspected tuberculosis and employees at a children's hospital. *Infect Control Hosp Epidemiol* 23:568–572, 2002.

13. Kellerman S.E., et al.: APIC and CDC survey of *Mycobacterium tuberculosis* isolation and control practices in hospitals caring for children. Part 1: Patient and family isolation policies and procedures. *Am J Infect Control* 26:478–482, Oct. 1998.

14. American Thoracic Society, Centers for Disease Control and Prevention, and Infectious Diseases Society of America: Treatment of tuberculosis. *MMWR Recomm Rep* 52:1–77, Jun. 20, 2003.

15. Centers for Disease Control and Prevention: Treating opportunistic infections among HIV-exposed and infected children: Recommendations from CDC, the National Institutes of Health, and the Infectious Diseases Society of America. *MMWR Recomm Rep* 53:1–100, Dec. 3, 2004.

16. Centers for Disease Control and Prevention: Tuberculosis transmission in multiple correctional facilities—Kansas, 2002–2003. *MMWR Morb Mortal Wkly Rep* 53:734–738, Aug. 20, 2004.

17. Centers for Disease Control and Prevention (CDC): *Reported Tuberculosis in the United States, 2003.* Atlanta: U.S. Department of Health and Human Services, CDC, Sep. 2004.

18. Centers for Disease Control and Prevention: Tuberculosis transmission in a homeless shelter population—New York, 2000–2003. *MMWR Morb Mortal Wkly Rep* 54:149–152, Feb. 18, 2005.

19. Centers for Disease Control and Prevention: Prevention and control of tuberculosis among homeless persons: Recommendations of the Advisory Council for the Elimination of Tuberculosis. *MMWR Recomm Rep* 41:1, Apr. 17, 1992.

20. Centers for Disease Control and Prevention: Recommendations for prevention and control of tuberculosis among foreign-born persons: Report of the Working Group on Tuberculosis Among Foreign-Born Persons. *MMWR Recomm Rep* 47:1–29, Sept. 18, 1998.

21. Centers for Disease Control and Prevention: Management of persons exposed to multidrug-resistant tuberculosis. *MMWR Recomm Rep* 41:59–71, Jun. 19, 1992.

Chapter 3

Infection Control

Because *Mycobacterium tuberculosis* is transmitted through the air and can sometimes take as long as days or weeks to diagnose correctly due to its vague and relatively common symptoms, stringent administrative, environmental, and respiratory protection controls are crucial to prevent the spread of the disease to health care workers and other patients in a health care facility. The following studies have shown that such precautions can significantly reduce the rate of tuberculosis transmission:

- A teaching hospital in New York City implemented the Centers for Disease Control and Prevention (CDC)'s 1994 guidelines for the prevention of tuberculosis transmission, including the following: (1) prompt isolation and treatment of patients with tuberculosis, (2) rapid diagnostic techniques for processing *M. tuberculosis* specimens, (3) negative-pressure isolation rooms, and (4) molded surgical masks for health care workers. As a result, the facility saw the proportion of patients with multidrug-resistant strains of *M. tuberculosis* drop from 32% to 14%. In addition, tuberculin skin test (TST) conversion rates for health care workers assigned to wards housing tuberculosis patients decreased from 17% to 5%, the same percentage as for health care workers assigned to other areas of the hospital.[1]
- Another New York hospital, which was the site of one of the first reported outbreaks of multidrug-resistant tuberculosis (MDR-TB) among acquired immune deficiency syndrome (AIDS) patients in the United States, implemented aggressive administrative, environmental, and infection controls over a four-year period. At the start of the three-phase study, 8.8% of AIDS patients hospitalized on the same ward on the same days as an infectious MDR-TB patient contracted the disease. During the second phase, that rate had dropped to 2.6%, and during the third phase, the facility had just one AIDS patient become infected with MDR-TB.[2]
- A hospital in Jacksonville, Florida, experienced an outbreak of MDR-TB among patients in its HIV ward, as well as an increase in TST conversions among its health care workers, and therefore decided to implement the CDC's 1994 guidelines. Before the controls recommended in the guidelines were put

into place, as many as 80% of MDR-TB patients had been exposed to another patient with the infection. After the controls were implemented, no episodes of MDR-TB could be traced to contact with infectious MDR-TB patients on the HIV ward. Before the controls, 28% of health care workers on the HIV ward had TST conversions; after the controls, none did.[3]

- At a university-affiliated urban hospital, expanded administrative controls reduced the number of tuberculosis exposure episodes (patients who were not placed in respiratory isolation at admission but who subsequently had a diagnosis of acid-fast bacilli [AFB] smear–positive pulmonary tuberculosis during that admission or within two weeks of discharge) decreased from 4.4 per month to 0.6 per month. TST conversion rates among health care workers declined from 3.3% to 0.4%.[4]

> Although standardized antituberculosis treatment regimens in the initial phase of therapy, rapid drug susceptibility testing, and directly observed therapy (DOT) have all helped diminish the number of people who contract and die from tuberculosis in its various forms, improvements in health care organizations' facilities, processes, and systems are vital to protecting patients and those who care for them from becoming infected in the first place.

As in the 1994 document, the CDC's 2005 guidelines emphasize the need for a defined program with controls designed to prevent the spread of tuberculosis. The recommendations are suggested for all health care settings to expedite rapid detection of tuberculosis, airborne precautions, and appropriate treatment or referral of patients who have suspected tuberculosis.

However, the recommendations differ somewhat, depending on whether an organization or setting regularly provides care or services to individuals who have or are suspected of having tuberculosis disease. The program, as defined in the guidelines, is based on a hierarchy of controls, starting with the overriding administrative controls, and then moving to environmental controls, and then respiratory protection controls.[5] The guidelines explain that the first two levels of controls (administrative and environmental) are used to minimize the number of areas in which exposure to *M. tuberculosis* might occur, and therefore minimize the number of persons exposed. Another expectation is that they will reduce (but not likely eliminate) the risk for exposure in areas where exposure does occur. The third level (respiratory protection controls) addresses the use of respiratory protective equipment in situations and areas that pose a high risk for exposure. Following are explanations of these controls and how implementing their recommendations can help a health care facility meet certain Joint Commission standards for infection controls and environmental controls (also *see* the Chapter 5 section, "Joint Commission International Standards").

Administrative Controls

Many people consider administrative controls to be the most important in reducing the risk of health care workers being exposed to patients who might have tuberculosis disease. Administrative controls involve the tasks of assigning responsibility for the tuberculosis infection control program, conducting the required risk assessment for the setting, and defining and implementing the infection control plan, as well as practices for managing patients. These controls require a program for training and educating health care workers about tuberculosis, as well as for screening and evaluating staff members who are at risk for tuberculosis or who might be exposed to patients with tuberculosis. They also include providing for necessary laboratory test processes and coordination with the local or state health departments.

Administrative controls, according to the CDC guidelines, consist of the following activities:
- Assigning responsibility for tuberculosis infection control in the health care setting
- Developing and instituting a written tuberculosis infection control plan to ensure prompt detection, airborne precautions, and treatment of persons who have suspected or confirmed tuberculosis disease
- Conducting a tuberculosis risk assessment of the setting
- Ensuring the timely availability of recommended laboratory processing, testing, and reporting of results to the ordering physician and infection control team
- Implementing effective work practices for the management of patients with suspected or confirmed tuberculosis disease
- Ensuring proper cleaning and sterilization or disinfection of potentially contaminated equipment (usually endoscopes)
- Training and educating health care workers regarding tuberculosis, with specific focus on prevention, transmission, and symptoms
- Screening and evaluating health care workers who are at risk for tuberculosis disease or who might be exposed to *M. tuberculosis* (for example, a tuberculosis screening program)

- Applying epidemiologic-based prevention principles, including the use of setting-related infection control data; using appropriate signage advising respiratory hygiene and cough etiquette
- Coordinating efforts with the local or state health department

Assigning Responsibility for Tuberculosis Infection Control and Developing an Infection Control Plan

Minimize Risk

The Joint Commission requires organizations to minimize the risk of a health care–associated infection through an organizationwide infection control (IC) program. This is measured by the following:

- All applicable organizational components and functions are integrated into the IC program.
- The organization has systems for reporting infection surveillance, prevention, and control information to the following:
  - The appropriate staff within the organization
  - Federal, state, and local public health authorities in accordance with law and regulation
  - Accrediting bodies
  - The referring or receiving organization where a patient was transferred or referred and the presence of an infection was not known at the time of transfer or referral
- Systems for the investigation of outbreaks of infectious diseases are in place.
- Applicable policies and procedures are in place throughout the organization.
- The organization has a written IC plan that includes the following:
  - A description of prioritized risks
  - A statement of the goals of the IC program
  - A description of the organization's strategies to minimize, reduce, or eliminate the prioritized risks
  - A description of how the strategies will be evaluated

Evaluate and Redesign

The Joint Commission requires organizations to ensure that the IC program evaluates the effectiveness of the IC interventions, and, as necessary, the organization redesigns the IC interventions. This is measured by the following:

- The organization formally evaluates and revises the goals and program (or portions of the program) at least annually and whenever risks significantly change.
- The evaluation addresses changes in the results of the IC program risk analysis.

- The evaluation addresses emerging and reemerging problems in the health care community that potentially affect the organization (for example, highly infectious agents).
- The evaluation addresses the assessment of the success or failure of interventions for preventing and controlling infection.
- The evaluation addresses the evolution of relevant infection prevention and control guidelines that are based on evidence or, in the absence of evidence, expert consensus.

Management

The Joint Commission requires the IC program to be effectively managed. This is measured by the following:

- The individual responsible for managing IC program activities coordinates all infection prevention and control activities within the organization.
- This individual facilitates ongoing monitoring of the effectiveness of prevention and/or control activities and interventions.

Collaboration

The Joint Commission requires that relevant components/functions within the organization collaborate to implement the IC program. This includes the following components/functions:

- Organization leaders, with licensed independent practitioners, medical staff, and other direct and indirect patient care staff (including, when applicable, administration, building maintenance/engineering, food services, housekeeping, laboratory, pharmacy, and sterilization services), collaborate on an ongoing basis with the qualified individual(s) managing the IC program.
- These representatives participate in the following:
  - Development of strategies for each component's/function's role in the IC program
  - Assessment of the adequacy of the human, information, physical, and financial resources allocated to support infection prevention and control activities
  - Assessment of the overall failure or success of key processes for preventing and controlling infection
  - The review and revision of the IC program as warranted to improve outcomes

Resource Management

The Joint Commission requires organization leaders to allocate adequate resources for the IC program. These activities are measured by the following:

- The effectiveness of the organization's infection prevention and control activities is reviewed on an ongoing basis, and findings are reported to the integrated patient safety program at least annually.
- Adequate systems to access information are provided to support infection prevention and control activities.
- Adequate laboratory support is provided to support infection prevention and control activities.
- Adequate equipment and supplies are provided to support infection prevention and control activities.

Monitor Environmental Conditions

The Joint Commission requires organizations to monitor conditions in the environment. These activities are measured by the following:

- The organization establishes and implements process(es) for reporting and investigating the following:
  - Injuries to patients/clients/residents or others coming to the organization's facilities, as well as incidents of property damage
  - Occupational illnesses and injuries to staff
  - Security incidents involving patients, staff, or others coming to the organization's facilities or property
  - Hazardous materials and waste spills, exposures, and other related incidents
  - Fire-safety management problems, deficiencies, and failures
  - Equipment management problems, failures, and user errors
  - Utility systems management problems, failures, or user errors
- The organization's leaders assign a person(s) to monitor and respond to conditions in the organization's environment. The assigned individuals performs the following tasks:
  - Coordinates the ongoing, organizationwide collection of information about deficiencies and opportunities for improvement in the environment of care
  - Coordinates the ongoing collection and dissemination of other sources of information, such as published hazard notices or recall reports
  - Coordinates the preparation of summaries of deficiencies, problems, failures, and user errors related to managing the environment of care
  - Coordinates the preparation of summaries on findings, recommendations, actions taken, and results of performance improvement activities
  - Participates in hazard surveillance and incident reporting
  - Participates in developing safety policies and procedures

Every health care facility should have an overall IC program that includes a tuberculosis infection control program. The CDC guidelines recommend that this program be based on whether the facility is one in which tuberculosis patients are likely to be encountered (for more on this distinction, *see* Chapter 1).

If the facility is one in which patients with suspected or confirmed tuberculosis are likely to be encountered, the CDC recommends the following:

1. Assign supervisory responsibility for the tuberculosis infection control program to a designated person or group with expertise in latent tuberculosis infection (LTBI) and tuberculosis disease, infection control, occupational health, environmental controls, and respiratory protection. This supervisor or supervisory body should have the support, authority, and specialized training to conduct a tuberculosis risk assessment, implement and enforce tuberculosis infection control policies, and ensure recommended training and education of health care workers. If it is a group that has supervisory responsibility, designate a single person (and a backup person) to whom questions can be directed.

2. Develop a written tuberculosis infection control plan that outlines a protocol for the prompt recognition of and initiation of airborne precautions for persons with suspected or confirmed tuberculosis disease, and update it annually (for more on identification and isolation of tuberculosis patients, *see* Chapter 2).

3. Conduct assessments (sometimes called problem evaluations) if a case of suspected or confirmed tuberculosis disease is not promptly recognized and appropriate airborne precautions not initiated, or if administrative, environmental, or respiratory protection controls fail.

4. Perform a contact investigation in collaboration with the local or state health department if health care–associated transmission of *M. tuberculosis* is suspected. Implement and monitor corrective action. (Contact investigations will be discussed in more detail later in this chapter.)

5. Collaborate with the local or state health department to develop administrative controls consisting of the risk assessment, written tuberculosis infection control plan, management of patients with suspected or confirmed tuberculosis disease, training and education of health care workers, screening and evaluation of health care workers, problem evaluation, and coordination.

6. Implement and maintain environmental controls, including airborne infection isolation (AII) room(s). (AII room(s) will be discussed in more detail later in this chapter.)

7. Implement a respiratory protection program (which will be discussed in more detail later in this chapter).
8. Perform ongoing training and education of health care workers. (For more on training and education, *see* Chapter 4.)
9. Create a plan for accepting patients who have suspected or confirmed tuberculosis disease if they are transferred from another setting.

If the facility is one in which patients with suspected or confirmed tuberculosis are *not* likely to be encountered, such patients will likely need to be transferred to a health care facility better equipped to diagnose and treat the illness effectively. The CDC recommends the following:

1. Assign responsibility for the tuberculosis infection control program to appropriate personnel.
2. Develop a written tuberculosis infection control plan that outlines a protocol for the prompt recognition and transfer of persons who have suspected or confirmed tuberculosis disease to another health care setting. The plan should indicate procedures to follow to separate persons with suspected or confirmed infectious tuberculosis disease from others until the time of transfer. Evaluate the plan annually, if possible, to ensure that the setting remains one in which persons who have suspected or confirmed tuberculosis disease are not likely to be encountered and that they are promptly transferred.
3. Conduct a problem evaluation if a case of suspected or confirmed tuberculosis disease is not promptly recognized, separated from others, and transferred.
4. Perform an investigation in collaboration with the local or state health department if health care–associated transmission of *M. tuberculosis* is suspected.
5. Collaborate with the local or state health department to develop administrative controls consisting of the risk assessment and the written tuberculosis infection control plan.

Conducting a Tuberculosis Risk Assessment of the Setting
Identifying Risk

The Joint Commission requires an IC program to identify risks for the acquisition and transmission of infectious agents on an ongoing basis. This is measured by the following:

• The organization identifies risks for the transmission and acquisition of infectious agents throughout the organization based on the following factors:

- The geographic location and community environment of the organization, program/services provided, and the characteristics of the population served
- The results of the analysis of the organization's infection prevention and control data
- The care, treatment, and services provided
- The risk analysis is formally reviewed at least annually and whenever significant changes occur in any of the above factors.
- Surveillance activities, including data collection and analysis, are used to identify infection prevention and control risks pertaining to the following:
  - Patients, clients, or residents
  - Licensed independent practitioners, staff, volunteers, and students/trainees
  - Visitors and families, as warranted

Priorities and Goals

Based on risks, The Joint Commission requires organizations to establish priorities and set goals for preventing the development of health care–associated infections within the organization. These activities are measured by the following:
- Priorities are established and goals related to preventing the acquisition and transmission of potentially infectious agents are developed based on the risks identified. These goals include, but are not limited to, the following:
  - Limiting unprotected exposure to pathogens throughout the organization

Emergency Management

As part of its emergency management activities, the Joint Commission requires organizations to have preparations to respond to an influx, or the risk of an influx, of infectious patients. These activities are measured by the following:
- The organization determines its response to an influx or risk of an influx of infectious patients.
- If the organization will continue to accept or treat patients, then the organization has a plan for managing an ongoing influx of potentially infectious patients over an extended period.
- The organization does the following:
  - Determines how it will keep abreast of current information about the emergency of epidemics or new infections that may result in the organization activating its response
  - Determines how it will disseminate critical information to staff and other key practitioners

Even if a facility does not seem likely to encounter a patient, client, or resident with suspected or confirmed tuberculosis, it is still vital that it perform a risk assessment. The assessment can help determine the types of controls that an organization needs to prevent the spread of tuberculosis and can also serve as a benchmark for comparison when risk assessments are conducted in the future.

– Identifies resources in the community (through local, state, and/or federal public health systems) for obtaining additional information

The CDC has separate sets of recommendations based on whether a facility is likely to encounter patients with suspected or confirmed tuberculosis. For organizations that *are* likely to see such patients, the recommendations are as follows:

1. Review the community profile of tuberculosis disease in collaboration with the state or local health department.
2. Consult the local or state tuberculosis control program to obtain epidemiologic surveillance data necessary to conduct a tuberculosis risk assessment.
3. Review the number of patients with suspected or confirmed tuberculosis disease who have been encountered in the facility during at least the previous five years.
4. Determine if persons with unrecognized tuberculosis disease have been admitted to or were encountered in the setting during the previous five years.
5. Determine which health care workers need to be included in a tuberculosis screening program and the frequency of screening required (tuberculosis screening for health care workers will be discussed later in this chapter).
6. Ensure the prompt recognition and evaluation of suspected episodes of health care–associated transmission of *M. tuberculosis* (for more on identification of tuberculosis patients, *see* Chapter 2).
7. Identify areas in the setting with an increased risk for health care–associated transmission of *M. tuberculosis* and target them for improved tuberculosis infection controls.
8. Assess the number of AII rooms needed for the setting. The risk classification for the setting should help to make this determination, depending on the number of tuberculosis patients examined. At least one AII room is needed for settings in which tuberculosis patients stay while being treated, and additional AII rooms might be needed, depending on the magnitude of patient-days of cases of suspect-

ed or confirmed tuberculosis disease. Additional AII rooms might be considered if options are limited for transferring patients with suspected or confirmed tuberculosis disease to other settings with AII rooms.

9. Determine the types of environmental controls needed other than AII rooms.
10. Determine which health care workers need to be included in the respiratory protection program.
11. Conduct periodic reassessments (annually, if possible) to ensure the following:
    - Proper implementation of the tuberculosis infection control plan
    - Prompt detection and evaluation of suspected tuberculosis cases
    - Prompt initiation of airborne precautions for suspected infectious tuberculosis cases
    - Recommended medical management of patients with suspected or confirmed tuberculosis disease
    - Functional environmental controls
    - Implementation of the respiratory protection program
    - Ongoing health care worker training and education regarding tuberculosis
12. Recognize and correct lapses in infection control.

For settings in which tuberculosis patients are not expected to be encountered, the CDC recommends the following:

1. Review the community profile of tuberculosis disease in collaboration with the local or state health department.
2. Consult the local or state tuberculosis control program to obtain epidemiologic surveillance data necessary to conduct a tuberculosis risk assessment.
3. Determine if persons with unrecognized tuberculosis disease were encountered in the setting during the previous five years.
4. Determine if any health care workers need to be included in the tuberculosis screening program (screening of health care workers will be discussed in more detail later in this chapter).
5. Determine the types of environmental controls that are currently in place and determine if any are needed in the setting.
6. Document procedures that ensure the prompt recognition and evaluation of suspected episodes of health care–associated transmission of *M. tuberculosis.*
7. Conduct periodic reassessments (annually, if possible) to ensure the following: (1) proper implementation of the tuberculosis infection control plan, (2) prompt detection and evaluation of suspected tuberculosis cases, (3) prompt initiation of airborne precautions for suspected infectious tuberculosis cases before transfer,

(4) prompt transfer of suspected infectious tuberculosis cases, (5) proper functioning of environmental controls, as applicable, and (6) ongoing tuberculosis training and education for health care workers.

8. Recognize and correct lapses in infection control.

The periodic assessments included in both sets of recommendations will help determine how well the tuberculosis infection control program is working and will identify any potential problems. This will also assist is correcting lapses in infection control practices. The CDC recommends reviewing the records of a sample of patients who had suspected or confirmed tuberculosis disease and were treated at the setting. The criteria or indicators suggested for review are as follows:

- Time interval from suspicion of tuberculosis until initiation of airborne precautions and antituberculosis treatment
- Time interval from suspicion of tuberculosis disease and patient triage to proper AII room or referral center for settings that do not provide care for patients with suspected or confirmed tuberculosis disease
- Time interval from admission until tuberculosis disease was suspected
- Time interval from admission until medical evaluation for tuberculosis disease was performed
- Time interval from admission until specimens for AFB smears and polymerase chain reaction–based nucleic acid amplification (NAA) tests for *M. tuberculosis* were ordered
- Time interval from admission until specimens for mycobacterial culture were ordered
- Time interval from ordering of AFB smears, NAA tests, and mycobacterial culture until specimens were collected
- Time interval from collection of specimens until performance and AFB smear results were reported
- Time interval from collection of specimens until performance and culture results were reported
- Time interval from collection of specimens until species identification was reported
- Time interval from collection of specimens until drug-susceptibility test results were reported
- Time interval from admission until airborne precautions were initiated
- Time interval from admission until antituberculosis treatment was initiated
- Duration of airborne precautions
- Measurement of meeting criteria for discontinuing airborne precautions; certain patients might be correctly discharged from an AII room to home

- Patient history of previous admission
- Adequacy of antituberculosis treatment regimens
- Adequacy of procedures for collection of follow-up sputum specimens
- Adequacy of discharge planning
- Number of visits to outpatient setting from the start of symptoms until tuberculosis disease was suspected (for outpatient settings)

Results of this review should be used to assess whether protocols need to be modified or retraining of staff members is required for the following:
- Prompt identification of possible tuberculosis disease and initiating airborne precautions
- Patient management
- Laboratory procedures

Implementing Effective Work Practices for the Management of Patients with Suspected or Confirmed Tuberculosis Disease
Specialized processes for handling patients suspected of or confirmed as having tuberculosis are vital to preventing transmission of the disease. Steps an organization can take to ensure that it has proper controls in place are discussed later in this chapter, as well as in Chapter 2.

Ensuring Proper Cleaning of Potentially Contaminated Equipment
Implementation
When the organization has prioritized it goals, the Joint Commission requires that strategies are implemented to achieve those goals. These activities are measured by the following:
- Methods to reduce the risks associated with procedures, medical equipment, and medical devices, including the following:
  - Appropriate storage, cleaning, disinfection, sterilization, and/or disposal of supplies and equipment
  - Reuse of equipment designated by the manufacturer as disposable in a manner that is consistent with regulatory and professional standards
  - The appropriate use of personal protective equipment
- Implementation of applicable precautions, as appopriate, is based on the following:
  - The potential for transmission
  - The mechanisms of transmission
  - The care, treatment, and service setting

– The emergence and reemergence of pathogens in the community that could affect the organization

Medical equipment and instruments used on tuberculosis patients are not frequently responsible for the transmission of the disease, but there have been some cases where *M. tuberculosis* was spread through a contaminated bronchoscope or other instrument introduced into the lungs. The following are examples in which the consequences of such contamination were extremely serious:

- A 1997 study by researchers from Johns Hopkins University School of Medicine found that a contaminated bronchoscope was likely the cause of transmission of *M. tuberculosis* from one patient (who was diagnosed with tuberculosis following the bronchoscopy) to another (who was diagnosed with small cell carcinoma following the bronchoscopy, and developed tuberculosis disease after six months of chemotherapy and radiation treatment).[6]
- In 1995 three people in South Carolina were found to have contracted MDR-TB when a bronchoscope previously used on another MDR-TB patient was not immersed in disinfectant, as it should have been, and was subsequently used on those three individuals.[7]
- After three patients at one hospital were found to have identical strains of tuberculosis, it was discovered that an atomizer used to apply lidocaine to the pharynx and nasal passages was not adequately disinfected and spread the disease from one patient to the other two.[8]
- In one case, the congenital form of the disease was spread from one premature infant to another through inadequately disinfected respiratory equipment.[9]

Decontamination of reusable medical equipment is always important, but the ease with which tuberculosis can be transmitted and the seriousness of the disease make decontamination particularly crucial. The following sections discuss CDC recommendations.

Critical Medical Instruments: Sterilization
Instruments such as surgical instruments, cardiac catheters, and implants, which are introduced directly into the bloodstream or other normally sterile areas of the body, must be sterilized before use.

Semicritical Medical Instruments: Sterilization or High-Level Disinfection
Instruments such as noninvasive flexible and rigid fiberoptic endoscopes or bronchoscopes, endotracheal tubes, and anesthesia breathing circuits, which might come into

contact with mucous membranes but ordinarily do not penetrate body surfaces, should be sterilized if possible. However, high-level disinfection that destroys vegetative microorganisms, the majority of fungal spores, mycobacteria (including tubercle bacilli), and small nonlipid viruses can be used.

High-level disinfection can be accomplished either manually or with an automated endoscope reprocessor with manual cleaning; however, manual cleaning is always the essential first step in the process to remove debris from the instrument.

Noncritical Medical Instruments or Devices: Disinfection
Instruments or devices such as crutches, bed boards, and blood pressure cuffs, which either do not ordinarily touch the patient or touch only the patient's intact skin, are not associated with transmission of *M. tuberculosis.* However, when this equipment is contaminated with blood or body substances, it should be cleaned and then disinfected with a hospital-grade, Environmental Protection Agency–registered germicide disinfectant with a label claim for tuberculocidal activity.

Tuberculocidal activity is not necessary for cleaning agents or low-level disinfectants that are used to clean or disinfect minimally soiled noncritical items and environmental surfaces (for example, floors, walls, tabletops, surfaces with minimal hand contact).

Training and Educating Health Care Workers Regarding Tuberculosis
The training and education of health care workers on tuberculosis prevention, symptoms, and transmission is a vital part of an infection control program. This topic is covered in more detail in Chapter 4.

Screening and Evaluating At-Risk Health Care Workers
Interventions
The Joint Commission requires that interventions are implemented that include the following:
- Screening for exposure and/or immunity to infectious diseases that licensed independent practitioners, staff, students/trainees, and volunteers may come in contact with in their work, as warranted
- Referral for assessment, potential testing, immunization and/or prophylaxis/treatment, and counseling, as appropriate, of licensed independent practitioners, staff, students/trainees, and volunteers who are identified as potentially having an infectious disease or risk of infectious disease that may put the population they serve at risk

- Referral for assessment, potential testing, immunization and/or prophylaxis/treatment, and counseling, as appropriate, of patients, students/trainees, and volunteers who have been exposed to infectious disease(s) at the hospital and licensed independent practitioners or staff who are occupationally exposed

Because of their close contact with a patient, client, or resident, health care workers are always at risk for contracting tuberculosis or other diseases from those they care for. The level of risk depends on the care setting, level of patient care responsibilities, prevalence of tuberculosis in the community, effectiveness of the facility's infection control program, and other factors, as noted in the following cases:

- A seven-year study of employees at the New York City Department of Health and Mental Hygiene found that 36.2% of U.S.-born employees in high-risk settings and 15.5% in low-risk settings were found to have baseline tuberculin positivity; the rate was 48.5% among employees born outside the U.S.[10]
- A 2005 study found that health care workers constitute more than 3% of tuberculosis cases in New York state.[11]
- A review of the database at the San Francisco Tuberculosis Control Section found that at least half of the cases of health care workers with tuberculosis were related to work.[12]
- A Japanese study found that 80% of nurses diagnosed with tuberculosis were likely to have contracted it through a nosocomial infection. However, about half of those were detected through mass tuberculosis screening of health care workers or contact tracing.[13]

Because of these risks and the importance of early treatment of tuberculosis, all health care workers—even those in settings considered to be low-risk, should receive a baseline tuberculosis screening.

Baseline Tuberculosis Screening
Screening health care workers for LTBI and tuberculosis disease at the beginning of employment. Tuberculosis screening includes a symptom screen for all health care workers, and TSTs or blood assay for *Mycobacterium tuberculosis* (BAMT) for those with previous negative test results for *M. tuberculosis* infection.

Health Care Workers Included in a Tuberculosis Surveillance Program

The definition of which health care workers are to be included in a surveillance program has been expanded from the 1994 version of the CDC guidelines. The 2005 definition includes the following:

- Paid and unpaid persons working in health care settings who have the potential for exposure to *M. tuberculosis* through shared air space with infectious patients
- Part-time, full-time, temporary, and contract staff
- All health care workers whose duties involve face-to-face contact with suspected or confirmed tuberculosis cases

In addition, health care workers who perform any of the following activities are to be included in the tuberculosis screening program:

- Entering patient, client, or resident rooms or treatment rooms whether or not the patient is present
- Participating in aerosol-generating or aerosol-producing procedures (for example, bronchoscopy, sputum induction, administration of aerosolized medications)
- Participating in suspected or confirmed *M. tuberculosis* specimen processing
- Installing, maintaining, or replacing environmental controls in areas where persons with tuberculosis are encountered

The conclusion then is that any health care worker who comes into contact with a known or suspected tuberculosis person, the spaces where they are housed or treated, or specimens that could possibly contain *M. tuberculosis* should be included in the surveillance program. Also included should be those who maintain, clean, and work with the environmental controls to ensure that they are working properly.

Another new element of the 2005 CDC guidelines is the risk classifications for health care workers and the fact that different levels and frequencies of testing are recommended for the different levels of risk.

A risk classification should usually be determined for an entire health care setting, but in some settings, such as large medical centers that include multiple care sites, types of services, communities, patient populations, and/or geographical regions, it may be reasonable to assign different risk classifications to different groups of health care workers. The 2005 CDC guidelines include examples of situations in which this might occur.

The following health care workers might be included in a tuberculosis screening program:

- Administrators or managers
- Bronchoscopy staff
- Chaplains
- Clerical staff
- Computer programmers
- Construction staff
- Correctional officers
- Craft or repair staff
- Dental staff
- Dietician or dietary staff
- Emergency department staff
- Engineers
- Food service staff
- Health aides
- Health and safety staff
- Homeless shelter staff
- Housekeeping or custodial staff
- Infection control staff
- Intensive care unit staff
- Janitorial staff
- Laboratory staff
- Maintenance staff
- Morgue staff
- Nurses
- Outreach staff
- Pathology laboratory staff
- Patient transport staff, including emergency medical service personnel
- Pediatric staff
- Pharmacists
- Physical and occupational therapists
- Physicians (assistants, attendings, fellows, residents, interns), including the following:
  – Anesthesiologists
  – Pathologists
  – Psychiatrists
  – Psychologists
- Public health educators or teachers
- Public safety staff
- Radiology staff
- Respiratory therapists
- Scientists
- Social workers
- Students (for example, medical, nursing, technicians, allied health)
- Technicians (for example, health, laboratory, radiology, animal)
- Veterinarians
- Volunteers

Tuberculosis Screening Risk Classifications

Low Risk. This classification should be applied to settings in which persons with suspected or confirmed tuberculosis disease are not expected to be encountered, because exposure to the bacterium is not likely. (Table 3-1, pages 95–96, provides more detail on how to determine risk classifications.) This classification should also be assigned to health care workers who will never have the opportunity to be exposed to patients with tuberculosis disease or to clinical specimens from such patients.

Screenings in this category should include the following:
- All health care workers should receive baseline tuberculosis screening upon hire, using two-step TST or a single blood assay for *Mycobacterium tuberculosis* (BAMT) to test for infection with *M. tuberculosis.*
- After baseline testing for infection with *M. tuberculosis,* additional tuberculosis screening is not necessary unless an exposure to *M. tuberculosis* occurs.
- Health care workers with a baseline of positive or a newly positive test result for *M. tuberculosis* infection (TST or BAMT), or documentation of treatment for LTBI or tuberculosis disease should receive one chest radiograph to exclude tuberculosis disease (or an interpretable copy within a reasonable time frame, such as six months). Repeat radiographs are not needed unless symptoms or signs of tuberculosis disease develop or unless recommended by a clinician.

Previously, all health care workers were required to have annual tuberculosis screenings; these recommendations represent a marked change, one that many low-risk facilities welcome. For example, a children's hospital in Kansas City, Missouri, which has been classified as low-risk, has been able to reduce the number of tuberculosis tests performed on health care workers from nearly 10,000 to 3,000 a year. This reduction will save the facility an estimated $50,000 a year. Other low-risk facilities still provide annual tuberculosis tests to those health care workers who want them, but those tests are no longer a requirement.[14]

Medium Risk. This classification should be applied to settings in which the risk assessment has determined that health care workers will or will possibly be exposed to persons with tuberculosis disease or to clinical specimens that might contain *M. tuberculosis.* If there is uncertainty as to whether a setting or group should be classified as low or medium risk, it should likely be classified as medium risk.

Screenings in this category should include the following:
- All health care workers should receive a baseline tuberculosis screening upon hire, using two-step TST or a single BAMT to test for infection with *M. tuberculosis.*
- After baseline testing for infection with *M. tuberculosis,* health care workers should receive tuberculosis screening annually (for example, symptom screen for all health care workers and testing for infection with *M. tuberculosis* for health care workers with baseline negative test results).
- Health care workers with a baseline positive or a newly positive test result for *M. tuberculosis* infection or documentation of previous treatment for LTBI or tubercu-

losis disease should receive one chest radiograph to exclude tuberculosis disease. Instead of participating in serial testing, health care workers should receive a symptom screen annually. This screen should be accomplished by educating the health care worker about symptoms of tuberculosis disease and instructing the health care worker to report any such symptoms immediately to the occupational health unit. Treatment for LTBI should be considered in accordance with CDC guidelines.

Potential Ongoing Transmission. This is a temporary risk classification, which should be applied to any setting or group of health care workers if there is evidence that *M. tuberculosis* has been transmitted from a patient or health care worker to another patient or health care worker in that setting during the preceding year. This evidence of person-to-person transmission includes the following:
1. Clusters or increased rates of TST or BAMT conversions
2. Health care workers with confirmed tuberculosis disease
3. Unrecognized tuberculosis disease in patients or health care workers
4. Recognition of an identical strain of *M. tuberculosis* in patients or health care workers with tuberculosis disease through DNA fingerprinting.

Screenings in this category should include the following:
- Testing for infection with *M. tuberculosis* might need to be performed every 8 to 10 weeks until lapses in infection control have been corrected and until no additional evidence of ongoing transmission is apparent.
- Classification of potential ongoing transmission should be used as a temporary classification only. It warrants immediate investigation and corrective steps. After a determination that ongoing transmission has ceased, the setting should be reclassified as medium risk. Maintaining the classification of medium risk for at least one year is recommended.

Health Care Workers Transferring Between Settings
When a health care worker transfers from one setting to another, even if the transfer is within the same organization, that person could be at a different level of risk for tuberculosis exposure in the new setting. In addition, a health care workers could potentially transfer between two settings that use different types of tuberculosis testing—for example, one might use TST whereas another uses BAMT. In these cases, a medical expert should review the different test results to make the necessary comparisons between the two.

Table 3-1. Guidelines for Low and Medium Risk Classifications

Risk determination is based on the number of tuberculosis patients encountered in the organization or setting within the previous year. Please note that Potential Ongoing Transmission *is not included because the definition of that classification is the same regardless of setting.*

Setting	Classification: Low	Classification: Medium
Inpatient: fewer than 200 beds	Fewer than three tuberculosis patients a year	Three or more tuberculosis patients a year
Inpatient: 200 or more beds	Fewer than six tuberculosis patients a year	Six or more tuberculosis patients a year
Outpatient settings and nontraditional facility-based settings: medical offices, ambulatory care centers, emergency medical services, long term care facilities	Fewer than three tuberculosis patients a year	Three or more tuberculosis patients a year
Emergency medical service, medical settings in correctional facilities, outreach care, long term care facilities	Only patients with LTBI treated No cough-inducing procedures are performed in setting. System to detect/triage persons with tuberculosis symptoms	Settings where tuberculosis patients are expected to be encountered
Correctional facilities		All correctional facilities should be classified as at least medium risk.

(continued)

Table 3-1. Guidelines for Low and Medium Risk Classifications, *continued*

Risk determination is based on the number of tuberculosis patients encountered in the organization or setting within the previous year. Please note that Potential Ongoing Transmission *is not included because the definition of that classification is the same regardless of setting.*

Setting	Classification: Low	Classification: Medium
Tuberculosis treatment facilities	Only patients with latent tuberculosis infections are treated. and No cough-inducing procedures are performed in the setting. and There is a defined system to detect and triage persons with tuberculosis symptoms.	Settings where tuberculosis patients are expected to be encountered
Laboratories	Laboratories in which clinical specimens that might contain *M. tuberculosis* are not manipulated.	Laboratories in which clinical specimens that might contain *M. tuberculosis* are manipulated.

Source: Centers for Disease Control and Prevention: Guidelines for preventing the transmission of *Mycobacterium tuberculosis* in health-care settings, 2005. *MMWR Recomm Rep* 54:1–147, Dec. 30, 2005.

Following are the CDC's recommendations for testing health care workers transferring to a new setting:

- When a health care worker transfers from one low-risk setting to another, a baseline result for infection with *M. tuberculosis* should be established and documented, after which serial testing is not necessary.
- When a health care worker transfers from a low-risk to a medium-risk setting, a baseline result for infection with *M. tuberculosis* should be established and documented. After that, annual tuberculosis screening (including a symptom screen and TST or BAMT for persons with previously negative test results) should be performed.
- When a health care worker transfers from a low- or medium-risk setting to a setting with a temporary classification of potential ongoing transmission, a baseline result for infection with *M. tuberculosis* should be established and documented. After that, a decision should be made regarding follow-up screening on an individual basis. If transmission seems to be ongoing, consider including the health care worker in the screenings every 8 to 10 weeks until a determination has been made that ongoing transmission has ceased. When the setting is reclassified back to medium risk, annual tuberculosis screening should be resumed.

Health Care Workers Who Test Positive

Health care workers with a baseline positive or newly positive test result (*see* Table 3-2, page 99) for *M. tuberculosis* infection should receive one chest radiograph result to exclude tuberculosis disease (or an interpretable copy within a reasonable time frame, such as six months).

Those who are determined to have LTBI do not pose a danger to patients or coworkers as they are not infectious, and therefore do not need to be removed from the workplace. These individuals should be encouraged to undergo treatment for LTBI, and should be educated about the risks of developing tuberculosis disease if LTBI is untreated. If a health care worker still chooses not to undergo treatment, he or she should not be removed from the workplace; however, that person should be educated about the symptoms of tuberculosis disease and instructed to report any such symptoms immediately to the occupational health unit. In addition, these health care workers should be informed that conditions that compromise the immune system, such as HIV, diabetes mellitus, certain cancers, and certain drug treatments, will increase the risk for rapid progression from LTBI to tuberculosis disease.

Health care workers who are found to have confirmed infectious pulmonary, laryngeal, endobroncheal, or tracheal tuberculosis disease, or a draining tuberculosis skin lesion pose a serious risk to patients, coworkers, and others. Those individuals should be excluded from the workplace until the following criteria have been met:

1. When they have had three negative AFB sputum smear results collected 8 to 24 hours apart, with at least one being an early morning specimen (because respiratory secretions pool overnight)
2. When they have responded to antituberculosis treatment that will probably be effective based on susceptibility results
3. When a physician that is knowledgeable and experienced in managing tuberculosis disease determines that the health care worker is noninfectious

Communicate with State and Local Authorities

Throughout the CDC guidelines are instructions to collaborate and consult with the local and state departments of health, in relation to the following:

- When planning and implementing tuberculosis control activities, these authorities can provide names of experts and other resources to help with policies, procedures, and program evaluation.
- When determining a setting's risk classification, health departments can provide data regarding the rates and epidemiology of tuberculosis within your community, and the type of client that uses your services.
- When you have a patient with suspected or confirmed tuberculosis disease, the local or state health department must be notified in accordance with law and regulation so that a community contact investigation can be conducted. The respective health department should be notified as early as possible and before the patient is discharged so that follow-up and continuation of therapy can be monitored by DOT. For inpatient settings, there should be discharge planning with the patient and the tuberculosis control program of the health department.

Environmental Controls

After administrative controls, the next line of defense against the transmission of tuberculosis is environmental controls. Environmental controls refer to the systems and processes designed to keep the health care environment—that is, patient rooms, examination rooms, and other areas of the facility—clean and free from *M. tuberculosis*. Because this bacterium is spread through the air, the most important environmental controls are those that prevent the spread and reduce the concentration of infectious droplet nuclei in the air. These include the following:

Table 3-2. Indications for Two-Step Tuberculin Skin Tests (TSTs)

Situation	Recommended testing
No previous TST result	Two-step baseline TSTs
Previous negative TST result (documented or not) >12 months before new employment	Two-step baseline TSTs
Previous documented negative TST result ≤12 months before new employment	Single TST needed for baseline testing; this test will be the second-step
≥2 previous documented negative TSTs but most recent TST >12 months before new employment	Single TST; two-step testing is not necessary
Previous documented positive TST result	No TST
Previous undocumented positive TST result*	Two-step baseline TST(s)
Previous BCG† vaccination	Two-step baseline TST(s)
Programs that use serial BAMT,§ including QFT¶ (or the previous version QFT)	See Supplement, Use of QFT-G** for Diagnosing *M. tuberculosis* Infections in Health-Care Workers (HCWs)

* For newly hired health-c are workers and other persons who will be tested on a routine basis (e.g., residents or staff of correctional or long-term–care facilities), a previous TST is not a contraindication to a subsequent TST, unless the test was associated with severe ulceration or anaphylactic shock, which are substantially rare adverse events. If the previous positive TST result is not documented, administer two-step TSTs or offer BAMT. **SOURCES:** Aventis Pasteur. Tuberculin purified protein derivative (Mantoux) Tubersol® diagnostic antigen. Toronto, Ontario, Canada: Aventis Pasteur; 2001. Parkdale Pharmaceuticals. APLISOL (Tuberculin purified protein derivative, diluted [stabilized solution]). Diagnostic antigen for intradermal injection only. Rochester, MI: Parkdale Pharmaceuticals; 2002. Froeschle JE, Ruben FL, Bloh AM. Immediate hypersensitivity reactions after use of tuberculin skin testing. Clin Infect Dis 2002;34:E12–3.
† Bacille Calmette-Guérin.
§ Blood assay for *Mycobacterium tuberculosis*.
¶ QuantiFERON®-TB test.
** QuantiFERON®-TB Gold test.

Source: Centers for Disease Control and Prevention, Department of Health and Human Services: Guidelines for preventing the transmission of *Mycobacterium tuberculosis* in health-care settings, 2005. *Morbidity and Mortality Weekly Report,* 2005; 54 (No. RR-17).

- Local exhaust ventilation
- General ventilation
- High-efficiency particulate air (HEPA) filtration
- Ultraviolet germicidal irradiation (UVGI; under limited conditions and as a supplement to other systems)

Local Exhaust Ventilation
Utility

The Joint Commission requires organizations to manage their utility risks. This is measured by the following activity:

- The organization designs, installs, and maintains ventilation equipment to provide appropriate pressure relationships, air exchange rates, and filtration efficiencies for ventilation systems serving areas specially designed to control airborne contaminants (such as biological agents, gases, fumes, and dust).

Utility Systems

The Joint Commission requires organizations to maintain, test, and inspect their utility systems. This is measured by the following:

- The organization maintains documentation of the maintenance of critical components of infection control utility systems/equipment for high-risk patients consistent with maintenance strategies identified in the utility management plan.

Local exhaust ventilation is a source-control technique used for capturing airborne contaminants (for example, infectious droplet nuclei or other infectious particles) before they are dispersed into the general environment. External hoods, enclosing booths, and tents are used in this technique. Local exhaust ventilation should be used when health care workers are inducing coughs in patients suspected of having tuberculosis or conducting any other procedure that can result in *M. tuberculosis* being released into the air (although this is not a substitute for personal respiratory protection, discussed later in this chapter).

General Ventilation

Managing Design and Building

The Joint Commission requires the organization to manage the design and building of the environment when it is renovated, altered, or newly created. This is measured by the following:

- When planning demolition, construction, or renovation, the organization conducts a proactive risk assessment using risk criteria to identify hazards that could potentially compromise care, treatment, and services in occupied areas of the organization's buildings. The scope and nature of the activities should determine the extent of risk assessment.
- When planning demolition, construction, or renovation, the organization uses risk criteria that address the impact of demolition, renovation, or new construction on air quality requirements, infection control, utility requirements, noise, vibration, and emergency procedures.

General ventilation systems are intended to remove contaminants from the air in a health care facility and to control the airflow patterns to prevent the spread of infection. The CDC guidelines recommend that a health care facility's engineering staff should include a professional with expertise in ventilation for health care settings; if this is not possible, a consultant with such expertise should be hired. This person should also be aware of all applicable federal, state, and local requirements as they relate to ventilation systems.

Sidebar 3-1.
Does Natural Ventilation Keep the Air Clean?

Research also shows that natural ventilation under ideal conditions—for example, opening windows and doors to let in fresh air—can be an effective, low-cost ventilation option. One study found that this method provided a median ventilation of 28 air changes per hour (ACH), more than double that of mechanically ventilated negative-pressure rooms ventilated at the 12 ACH recommended for high-risk areas. Researchers also discovered that facilities built more than 50 years ago, which generally have higher ceilings and larger windows, had better ventilation than more modern buildings. While natural ventilation is not always possible in large, multistory medical facilities, it can be an excellent option for smaller facilities (climate permitting) that cannot afford the cost of installing and maintaining a mechanical ventilation system.

Source: Escombe A.R., et al.: Natural ventilation for the prevention of airborne contagion. *PloS Med* 4:309–316, Feb. 2007.

In some facilities, natural ventilation can be an effective and viable option. *See* Sidebar 3-1 for more information.

AII rooms in existing health care settings should have airflow of at least 6 ACH, with the option to increase the airflow to at least 12 ACH by adjusting the ventilation system or by using air-cleaning methods such as HEPA filters or UVGI systems. When buildings are renovated or newly constructed, ventilation systems should be designed so that AII rooms have airflow of at least 12 ACH. Tables 3-3 and 3-4, pages 102 and 103, respectively, provide more data on the number of ACH required to clean the air effectively.

Air Changes per Hour (ACH)
Air change rate expressed as the number of air exchange units per hour.

Table 3-3. Air Changes per Hour (ACH) and Time Required to
Remove Most Air Contaminants

This table can be used to estimate the time necessary to clear the air of airborne Mycobacterium tuberculosis *after the source patient leaves the area or when aerosol-producing procedures are complete.*

ACH	Minutes required for removal efficiency*	
	99%	99.9%
2	138	207
4	69	104
6	46	69
12	23	35
15	18	28
20	7	14
50	3	6
400	< 1	1

* Time in minues to reduce the airborne concentration by 99% or 99.9%.

Source: Centers for Disease Control and Prevention: Guidelines for preventing the transmission of *Mycobacterium tuberculosis* in health-care settings, 2005. *MMWR Recomm Rep* 54:1–147, Dec. 30, 2005.

HEPA Filtration

HEPA filters can be used to filter infectious droplet nuclei from the air. They must be used (1) when discharging air from local exhaust ventilation booths or enclosures directly into the surrounding room or area, and (2) when discharging air from an AII room (or other negative-pressure room) into the general ventilation system (for example, in settings in which the ventilation system or building configuration makes venting the exhaust to the outside impossible). HEPA filters can also be used as a safety measure in exhaust ducts to remove droplet nuclei from air being discharged to the outside. The HEPA filters must be installed at the inlet of exhaust to prevent duct contamination by nuclei.

Air can be recirculated through HEPA filters in areas in which (1) no general venti-lation system is present, (2) in which an existing system is incapable of providing suf-

Table 3-4. Ventilation Recommendations for Certain Health Care Settings

Health-care setting	Minimum mechanical ACH*	Minimum outdoor ACH*	Air movement relative to adjacent areas	Air exhausted directly outdoors†
Microbiology laboratory	6	§	In	Yes
Anteroom to AII¶ room	10	§	In/Out	Yes
AII room**††	12	2	In	Yes
Autopsy suite	12	§	In	Yes
Bronchoscopy room	12	2	In	Yes
Emergency department and radiology waiting rooms	12–15§§	2	In	Yes
Operating room or surgical room	15¶¶	3§§	Out	§
	25***	15¶¶		
		5***		

SOURCES: CDC. Guidelines for preventing the transmission of *Mycobacterium tuberculosis* in health-care facilities, 1994. MMWR 1994;43(No. RR-13). American Society of Heating, Refrigerating, and Air-Conditioning Engineers, Inc. Health care facilities [Chapter 7]. 2003 ASHRAE handbook: HVAC applications. Atlanta, GA: American Society of Heating, Refrigerating, and Air-Conditioning Engineers, Inc.; 2003: 7.1-7.14

* Air changes per hour.

† If it is not possible to exhaust all the air to the outdoors in existing or renovated facilities, the air can be recirculated after passing through high efficiency particulate air (HEPA) filtration.

§ American National Standards Institute (ANSI/American Society of Heating, Refrigerating, and Air-Conditioning Engineers, Inc. (ASHRAE). Standard 62.1-2004. Ventilation for Acceptable Indoor Air Quality, should be consulted for outside air recommendations in areas that are not specified. SOURCE: ANSI/ASHRAE. Standard 62.1-2004-ventilation for acceptable indoor air quality. Atlanta, GA: ASHRAE; 2004.

¶ Airborne infection isolation.

** Settings with existing All rooms should have an airflow of ?6 mechanical ACH; air-cleaning devices can be used to increase the equivalent ACH.

†† Patients requiring a protective environment room (e.g., severely immunocompromised patients) who also have TB disease require protection from common airborne infectious microorganisms.

§§ Recommendation of the American Institute of Architects (AIA) (air is recirculated through HEPA filters). Source: AIA. Guidelines for design and construction of hospital and health care facilities. Washington, DC: AIA; 2001.

¶¶ Recommendation of ASHRAE (100% exhaust). Source: ANSI/ASHRAE. Standard 62.1-2004-ventilation for acceptable indoor air quality. Atlanta, GA: ASHRAE; 2004.

*** Recommendation of ASHRAE (air is recirculated through HEPA filters). SOURCE: ANSI/ASHRAE. Standard 62.1-2004. Atlanta, GA: ASHRAE; 2004.

Source: Centers for Disease Control and Prevention: Guidelines for preventing the transmission of *Mycobacterium tuberculosis* in health-care settings, 2005. *MMWR Recomm Rep* 54:1–147, Dec. 30, 2005.

ficient ACH, or (3) in which air-cleaning without affecting the fresh-air supply or negative-pressure system is desired. Such uses can supplement the number of equivalent ACH in the room or area.

Although particulates in the air will eventually disperse on their own due to the facility's general ventilation system, waiting for this to occur is not possible in today's health care environment. Rooms that have been vacated need to be cleaned and available to new patients as soon as possible, and HEPA filters help in that regard. One study found that in unfiltered rooms, it took a minimum of 171 minutes for 90% of aerosolized contaminants to be removed, whereas portable HEPA filters were able to remove 90% of contaminants in 5 to 31 minutes.[15] This rapid cleaning of the air not only makes rooms available to new patients, but significantly decreases the possibility that a patient or health care worker would be inadvertently exposed to *M. tuberculosis.*

Ultraviolet Germicidal Irradiation

UVGI is a supplemental air-cleaning technology that can be used in a room or corridor to irradiate the air in the upper portion of the room. It is installed in a duct to irradiate air passing through the duct or is incorporated into room air-recirculation units; it can be used in ducts that recirculate air back into the same room or in ducts that exhaust air directly to the outside.

However, UVGI *should not* be used in place of HEPA filters when discharging air from isolation booths or enclosures directly into the surrounding room or area or when discharging air from an AII room into the general ventilation system. This is because effective use of UVGI ensures that infectious droplets of *M. tuberculosis* are exposed to a sufficient dose of ultraviolet-C to result in inactivation. Because this is based on time as well as irradiance, the effectiveness of any application is determined by its ability to deliver sufficient irradiance for enough time to result in inactivation of the organism within the infectious droplet. Achieving a sufficient dose can be difficult with airborne inactivation because the exposure time can be substantially limited; therefore, attaining sufficient irradiance is essential.

Respiratory Protection Controls

Administrative and environmental controls are meant to minimize the number of areas in which exposure to *M. tuberculosis* might occur and, therefore, to minimize the number of persons exposed. However, although these controls reduce the risk for exposure in the limited areas in which exposure can occur, they do not eliminate that risk. Therefore, persons entering these areas might be exposed to *M. tuberculosis*. Respiratory protection controls further protect health care workers and others in situations that pose a high risk for exposure.

Respiratory protection controls include implementing a respiratory protection program, training health care workers on respiratory protection, and training patients on respiratory hygiene and cough etiquette procedures (the importance of turning their heads away from persons and covering their mouths and noses with their hands—or preferably with a cloth or tissue—when coughing or sneezing).

The CDC guidelines provide directions regarding persons who should use respiratory protective equipment, including the following:
- All persons, including health care workers and visitors, entering rooms where patients with suspected or confirmed infectious tuberculosis disease are being isolated
- Persons present during cough-inducing or aerosol-generating procedures performed on patients with suspected or confirmed infectious tuberculosis disease
- Persons in other settings in which administrative and environmental controls will probably not protect them from inhaling infectious airborne droplet nuclei, such as those who transport patients with suspected or confirmed infectious tuberculosis disease and those who provide urgent surgical or dental care to such patients
- In addition, laboratory staff conducting aerosol-producing procedures might require respiratory protection.

The following criteria need to be met by respiratory protective equipment used in health care settings:
- They must be certified by the CDC/National Institute for Occupational Safety and Health (NIOSH) as a nonpowered particulate filter respirator (N-, R-, or P-95, 99, or 100), including disposable respirators or powered air-purifying respirators (PAPRs) with high-efficiency filters.
- They must be able to adequately fit respirator wearers (for example, a fit factor of greater than 100 for disposable and half-mask respirators) who are included in a respiratory protection program.
- They must be able to fit the different facial sizes and characteristics of health care workers.

Powered Air-Purifying Respirator (PAPR)
A respirator equipped with a tight-fitting facepiece (rubber facepiece) or loose-fitting facepiece (hood or helmet), breathing tube, air-purifying filter, cartridge or canister, and fan. Air is drawn through the air-purifying element and pushed through the breathing tube and into the facepiece, hood, or helmet by the fan. Loose-fitting PAPRs (for example, hoods or helmets) might be useful for persons with facial hair because they do not require a tight seal with the face.

Assistance with the selection of respirators can be obtained through consultation with the CDC, respirator fit-testing experts, occupational health and infection control organizations, and respirator manufacturers and through peer-reviewed research and advance respirator training courses. It is important to note that surgical masks are *not* sufficient protection against infectious airborne particles, including tuberculosis and influenza.[16]

Respirator Options

N95 masks, one of the most commonly used types of respirators, have been certified by the NIOSH to be at least 95% effective at filtering out airborne particles of 0.3 microns or larger. The airborne droplet nuclei containing *M. tuberculosis* are 0.5 microns or larger, and the N95 mask will prevent the wearer from inhaling them. The N95 mask provides the minimum level of protection for health care workers.

However, there may be special circumstances in which respiratory protective devices that exceed the minimum level provided by an N95 respirator may be desirable. Such circumstances might include bronchoscopy or autopsy procedures on persons with suspected or confirmed tuberculosis disease and selected laboratory procedures. Additional protection can be provided by full-facepiece respirators or PAPRs. In addition, in cases in which health care workers are at risk for both inhalation exposure to *M. tuberculosis* and mucous membrane exposure to bloodborne pathogens, a nonfluid-resistant respirator with a full-face shield or a combination product surgical mask/N95 disposable respirator could be used to achieve protection from both pathogen sources. The CDC guidelines provide a supplement that includes more detail on the types of respirators and the circumstances in which they should be used. Table 3-5, page 107, also provides guidance as to the types of respirators that are best for different settings.

Table 3-5. Settings Where the Use of Personal Respiratory Protection Is Most Likely to Prevent Occupational Tuberculosis

Setting	Estimated dissemination rate (infectious units per hour)	Recommended respirator	Comments
Autopsies	> 1,000	PAPR hood*	Highest risk probably associated with the creation of aerosols by bone saws
Bronchoscopy and endotracheal intubation	25,035	PAPR hood*	Possibly high risk due to induction of cough and dilution of mucous with saline
Laryngeal tuberculosis	6,038	N95[†]	Possibly high risk due to increased strength and frequency of cough
Cavitary tuberculosis (untreated)	1,339	N95[†]	Higher bacillary load in cavities compared to nodules or infiltrates
Tuberculosis ward with patients receiving appropriate drug therapy	1.2538 (average)	N95[†] to none	Risk decreases with treatment and with appropriate room ventilation

* PAPR hood, powered air-purifying respirator hood.
[†] N95, disposable particulate respirator equivalent to the U.S. NIOSH N95 class.

Sources: Fennelly, K.P.: The role of masks in preventing nosocomial transmission of tuberculosis. *Int J Tuberc Lung Dis* 2:S103–S109, 1998.
Catanzaro A.: Nosocomial tuberculosis. *American Review of Respiratory Disease* 125:559–562, 1982.
Fennelly K.P., Nardell E.A.: The relative efficacy of respirators and room ventilation in preventing occupational tuberculosis. *Infect Control Hosp Epidemiol* 19:754–759, Oct. 1998.
Nardell E.A., et al.: Airborne infection: Theoretical limits of protection achievable by building ventilation. *American Review of Respiratory Disease* 144:302–306, 1991.
Riley R.L., et al.: Infectiousness of air from a tuberculosis ward—Ultraviolet irradiation of infected air: Comparative infectiousness of different patients. *American Review of Respiratory Disease* 85:511–525, 1962.
Templeton G.L., et al.: The risk of transmission of *Mycobacterium tuberculosis* at the bedside and during autopsy. *Ann Intern Med* 122:922–925, 1995.

Fit Testing

If a respirator does not fit snugly on the face, infectious airborne droplets could potentially be inhaled around the sides of the mask. This is why fit testing is so important.[16,17] A fit test is used to determine which respirator fits the user adequately and to assess whether the user knows when the respirator is fitting properly. Fit testing should be performed in the initial training for respiratory protection and periodically thereafter.

The two types of fit testing are quantitative or qualitative. Because everyone's face is different, there is no way to ensure a proper fit for a face mask without this type of direct testing. Quantitative fit testing requires a tester to count the particles outside and inside the respirator; qualitative fit testing measures the ability of the wearer to smell or taste particles from an aerosol spray. Both types of testing have their challenges, however: One study found that one in five respirator wearers may pass a fit test in error.[18]

The frequency with which fit testing should occur is a topic of some disagreement in the health care field. While the Occupational Safety and Health Administration (OSHA) requires annual fit testing, the CDC guidelines simply recommend "periodic" testing. Many experts believe that annual fit testing is vital to health care worker safety—this regulation is supported by the CDC, the NIOSH, the Institute of Medicine, and the American Nurses Association (ANA), for example—but others say that this is a waste of time and resources.

In previous years, Rep. Roger Wicker (R-Missouri) has attached a rider to appropriations legislation that would prohibit OSHA from enforcing the annual fit-test requirement. Rep. Wicker says that the fit-testing requirement is too burdensome and that the decline in tuberculosis cases over the last few years has made it unnecessary. The ANA, however, notes that fit-tested respirators protect health care workers from severe acute respiratory syndrome (SARS), avian flu, influenza, and anthrax in addition to tuberculosis, and cites a recent case in which a nurse died after contracting tuberculosis due to an improperly fitted respirator. The organization also says that fit testing costs hospitals an average of just $16.80 per year.[19,20]

At the CDC Workshop on Respiratory Protection for Airborne Infectious Agents, held in late 2004, physicians, industrial hygiene professionals, and other experts had widely differing opinions on the subject. However, many agreed that a possible solution would be to develop different sets of fit-testing requirements based on a health care setting's tuberculosis risk classification.

The CDC suggests that the frequency of fit testing be determined by the occurrence of (1) risk for transmission of *M. tuberculosis,* (2) a change in facial features of the wearer, (3) a medical condition that would affect respiratory function, (4) physical characteristics of the respirator (despite the same model number), or (5) a change in the model or size of the assigned respirator. Organizations developing fit-testing plans should stay abreast of the latest updates and regulations.

References

1. Maloney S.A., et al.: Efficacy of control measures in preventing nosocomial transmission of multidrug-resistant tuberculosis to patients and health care workers. *Ann Intern Med* 122:90–95, Jan. 15, 1995.

2. Stroud L.A., et al.: Evaluation of infection control measures in preventing the nosocomial transmission of multidrug-resistant *Mycobacterium tuberculosis* in a New York City hospital. *Infect Control Hosp Epidemiol* 16:141–147, Mar. 1995.

3. Wenger P.N., et al.: Control of nosocomial transmission of multidrug-resistant *Mycobacterium tuberculosis* among healthcare workers and HIV–infected patients. *Lancet* 345:235–240, Jan. 28, 1995.

4. Blumberg H.M.: Preventing the nosocomial transmission of tuberculosis. *Ann Intern Med* 122:658–663, May 1, 1995.

5. Centers for Disease Control and Prevention: Guidelines for preventing the transmission of *Mycobacterium tuberculosis* in health-care settings. *MMWR Recomm Rep* 54:1–147, Dec. 30, 2005.

6. Michele T.M., et al.: Transmission of *Mycobacterium tuberculosis* by a fiberoptic bronchoscope: Identification by DNA fingerprinting. *JAMA* 278:1093–1095, Oct. 1, 1997.

7. Agerton T., et al.: Transmission of a highly drug-resistant strain (strain W1) of *Mycobacterium tuberculosis:* Community outbreak and nosocomial transmission via a contaminated bronchoscope. *JAMA* 278:1073–1077, Oct. 1, 1997.

8. Southwick K.L., et al.: Cluster of tuberculosis cases in North Carolina: Possible association with atomizer reuse. *Am J Infect Control* 29:1–6, Feb. 2001.

9. Crockett M., et al.: Nosocomial transmission of congenital tuberculosis in a neonatal intensive care unit. *Clin Infect Dis* 39:1719–1723, Dec. 1, 2004.

10. Cook S., et al.: Prevalence of tuberculin skin test positivity and conversions among healthcare workers in New York City during 1994 to 2001. *Infect Control Hosp Epidemiol* 24:807–813, Nov. 2003.

11. Driver C.R., et al.: Tuberculosis in health care workers during declining tuberculosis incidence in New York State. *Am J Infect Control* 33:519–526, Nov. 2005.

12. Ong A., et al.: Tuberculosis in healthcare workers: A molecular epidemiologic study in San Francisco. *Infect Control Hosp Epidemiol* 27:453–458, May 2006.

13. Ohmori M., et al.: Current epidemiological situation of tuberculosis in the workplace: Considering the risk of tuberculosis among nurses. *Kekkaku [Tuberculosis]* 82:85–93, Feb. 2007.

14. Freedom: Hospitals halt annual TB tests. *Hospital Employee Health,* Aug. 1, 2006.

15. Rutala W.A., et al.: Efficacy of portable filtration units in reducing aerosolized particles in the size range of *Mycobacterium tuberculosis. Infect Control Hosp Epidemiol* 16:391–398, Jul. 1995.

16. Lawrence R.B., et al.: Comparison of performance of three different types of respiratory protection devices. *J Occup Environ Hyg* 3:465–474, Sep. 2006.

17. Fay S., Narayan M.C.: Diagnosis: Tuberculosis. *Home Healthc Nurse* 24:236–246, Apr. 2006.

18. Coffey C.C., et al.: Errors associated with three methods of assessing respirator fit. *J Occup Environ Hyg* 3:44–52, Jan. 2006.

19. McKeon E.: 109th adjourns without action on funding: Wicker rider remains. *Capitol Update* 4, Dec. 22, 2006. http://www.capitolupdate.org/Newsletter/index.asp?nlid=188& nlaid=812 (accessed Oct. 4, 2007).

20. McKeon E.: The ANA champions respiratory protections for nurses. *Am J Nurs* 106:31, Jun. 2006.

Chapter 4

Patient, Visitor, and Health Care Worker Education

One of the greatest tools we have in the fight against the spread of tuberculosis is education. Information on how the disease is transmitted, detected, treated, and prevented can help patients, their families, and health care workers all take the necessary precautions to keep the incidence of tuberculosis at bay. The following sections discuss steps a health care organization can take to ensure that these groups receive the appropriate information about tuberculosis.

Health Care Staff Education

Anyone who may come in contact with infectious patients—including not only health care workers but also other hospital workers, such as housekeepers, volunteers, students, engineers—should be educated about reducing disease transmission risks. Health care workers whose positions put them at particularly high risk of exposure to *Mycobacterium tuberculosis* need training on how to protect themselves, their patients, and others in addition to their education on the diagnosis and treatment of tuberculosis, as well as the health care facility's procedures regarding tuberculosis. Training and education of health care workers will not only inform them of the organization's infection control program—it will also increase adherence to the program's protocols.

Because health care workers receive many types of training, it can be beneficial to combine tuberculosis training with training for other types of infectious diseases, such as severe acute respiratory syndrome (SARS) because many infection control protocols will be similar. However, health care facilities should ensure that those issues that are specific to tuberculosis are also addressed.

Patient Education

When a person has been diagnosed with latent tuberculosis infection (LTBI) or tuberculosis, it is vital that the person be made to understand the importance of obtaining proper treatment and the seriousness of the consequences if he or she chooses not to. Health care workers working with tuberculosis patients need to be

Patients also need to be made aware of how the disease is transmitted and how they can reduce risks to others. Risk reduction strategies include respiratory hygiene and cough etiquette procedures—that is, turning their heads away from others and covering their mouths and noses with their hands, a cloth, or a tissue when coughing or sneezing—and to keeping isolation room doors closed when necessary.

aware that some groups that tend to be at risk for tuberculosis, particularly the homeless, drug users, and prisoners, may have some resistance to following instructions from an authority figure; they also might be unwilling or unable to provide some of the personal information and medical history needed to initiate a contact investigation. In these cases, health care workers will need to exert some effort in not only educating patients, but also in earning their trust and confidence. In fact, studies have shown that emotional support from nurses can have a positive effect on health outcomes for tuberculosis patients.[1]

Although health care workers who provide direct patient care—particularly, physicians, nurses, and respiratory therapists—are the primary source of tuberculosis patient education, pharmacists can also play a vital role in educating patients about how their treatment will work and about the importance of continuing it until their physician determines that they are tuberculosis-free. In fact, one study found that when patients received pharmacist-directed education about their condition and treatment, they were nearly twice as likely to attend all of their required hospital visits. The education consisted of written and oral material: The written material was an illustrated handout designed in question-and-answer format, with material reviewed by physicians and laypeople to ensure accuracy as well as readability; the oral material was a summary of the key points mentioned in the written material. An additional handout with detailed information about proper drug use was also included.[2]

Printed handouts or brochures that patients can take home for later reference can be helpful in this process. The Centers for Disease Control and Prevention (CDC) have numerous resources available to help educate patients about their condition. The "Education/Training Materials" area of the CDC Web site includes a list of pamphlets that you can either download in PDF format or order from the CDC. The list can be found at http://www.cdc.gov/tb/pubs/pamphlets.htm and includes such titles as *Get the Facts About TB Disease, Protect Your Family and Friends from TB: The Contact Investigation, Staying on Track with TB Medicine,* and *Take Steps to Control TB When You Have HIV.* A booklet of frequently asked questions (FAQs) is also available from the CDC at http://www.cdc.gov/tb/faqs/pdfs/qa.pdf. (*See* Figure 4-1, pages 114–115, for sample pages from the FAQ booklet.)

These publications include vital information about tuberculosis in an easy-to-read and easy-to-understand format. Be aware, however, that it is not enough to simply distribute these materials to patients; health care workers should be prepared to review the information with patients and answer questions.

The CDC also offers the *TB Education and Training Resources* Web site (http://www.findtbresources.org), where other organizations can share their tuberculosis-related educational materials. The database includes materials submitted from a variety of community and racial/ethnic organizations to help communicate with the various patient populations served. *See* Figure 4-2, pages 116–117, for examples (also, *see* Sidebar 4-1 later in this chapter for more information on this and other online training resources).

Visitor and Family Education

Visitors and family members need to know their risks of becoming infected and what measures they can take to protect themselves. Conversely, close contacts, particularly parents and family members of children with tuberculosis, may have transmitted the disease to the patient and may require evaluation, isolation, and treatment.[3] For example, researchers at Texas Children's Hospital tested the caretakers of 59 children brought to the hospital with tuberculosis and found that 15% of them had previously undetected pulmonary tuberculosis. In all of the cases in which the adult was the child's parent and caretaker, that person was the source of the child's infection.

Contact Investigations

After a patient has been diagnosed with tuberculosis disease, a contact investigation can help prevent further spread of the disease by identifying the person from whom the patient contracted tuberculosis, as well as any others to whom the patient might have inadvertently spread the disease. These individuals can be tested and, if necessary, receive treatment. They can also be educated about tuberculosis and its transmission so they can protect themselves from infection and recognize symptoms if they do occur.

Figure 4-1. **Sample Pages from *Questions and Answers About Tuberculosis (TB)***

LATENT TB INFECTION

How can I get tested for TB?

You should get tested for TB if
*   You have spent time with a person known to have active TB disease or suspected to have active TB disease; or

*   You have HIV infection or another condition that puts you at high risk for active TB disease; or

*   You think you might have active TB disease; or

*   You are from a country where active TB disease is very common (most countries in Latin America and the Caribbean, Africa, Asia, Eastern Europe, and Russia); or

*   You live somewhere in the United States that active TB disease is more common such as a homeless shelter, migrant farm camp, prison or jail, and some nursing homes; or

*   You inject illegal drugs.

The TB skin test

The TB skin test may be used to find out if you have TB infection. You can get a skin test at the health department or at your doctor's office. A health care worker will inject a small amount of testing fluid (called tuberculin or PPD) just under the skin on the under side of the forearm. After 2 or 3 days, you must return to have your skin test read by the health care worker. You may have a swelling where the tuberculin was injected. The health care worker will measure this

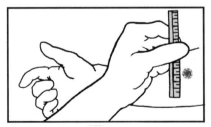

Q & A About TB   5

(continued)

Figure 4-1. **Sample Pages from *Questions and Answers About Tuberculosis (TB), continued***

ACTIVE TB DISEASE

How is active TB disease treated?

There is good news for people with active TB disease! It can almost always be cured with medicine. But the medicine must be taken as the doctor or nurse tells you.

If you have active TB disease, you will need to take several different medicines. This is because there are many bacteria to be killed. Taking several medicines will do a better job of killing all of the bacteria and preventing them from becoming <u>resistant</u> to the medicines.

The most common medicines used to cure TB are

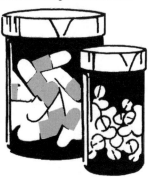

- isoniazid (INH)
- rifampin (RIF)
- ethambutol
- pyrazinamide

If you have active TB disease of the lungs or throat, you are probably infectious. You need to stay home from work or school so that you don't spread TB bacteria to other people. After taking your medicine for a few weeks, you will feel better and you may no longer be infectious to others. Your doctor or nurse will tell you when you can return to work or school or visit with friends.

Having active TB disease should not stop you from leading a normal life. When you are no longer infectious or feeling sick, you can do the same things you did before you had active TB disease. The medicine that you are taking should not affect your strength, sexual function, or ability to work. If you take your medicine as your doctor or nurse tells you, the medicine will kill all the TB bacteria. This will keep you from becoming sick again.

Q & A About TB   9

Source: Centers for Disease Control and Prevention: *Questions and Answers About TB.* 2005. http://www.cdc.gov/tb/faqs/pdfs/qa.pdf (accessed Jul. 12, 2007).

Figure 4-2. Sample Resources from the CDC's TB Education and Training Resources Web Site

Patient Brochure from the County of San Diego Health and Human Services Agency

- Keep your medicine in a place where you cannot miss it.

  Try keeping your bottle in the bathroom or in the kitchen, anywhere a glass of water is handy.

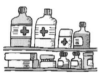

** *As with all medicine, make sure all your TB medicine is out of reach of children.* ******

You can lead a normal life.

Remember, unless you have TB disease, you are not sick. You are taking medication to prevent you from getting sick. Don't be afraid to be with people. Work, exercise, and socialize like you normally do. You can't give TB to others unless you have disease.

A word to parents:

If you are the parent of a child who has TB infection (not disease), the same facts apply to your child. Let your child play with others and go to school.

Things to watch for:

Treatment for TB infection is safe for most people. But, like any medicine, INH and other medicines used to treat TB infection can sometimes have side effects. Ask your doctor what to look for. Some things to watch for include:

- Tiredness
- Nausea
- Loss of appetite
- Easy bruising or bleeding
- Flu-like symptoms
- Vomiting
- Rash
- Stomach or abdominal pain
- Joint aches
- Other problems that concern you

** *If you have side effects, STOP taking the pills and call your doctor or clinic* ******

County of San Diego
Health and Human Services Agency
3851 Rosecrans Street, P.O. Box 85222
San Diego, CA 92186-5222
(619) 692-8800
www.sandiegotbcontrol.org

You may qualify for Medi-Cal benefits.
People with TB infection or TB disease may also qualify for TB-Cal. To find out about your eligibility and to request an information packet and application, please call 1-858-514-6885. Collect calls are accepted.

HHSA:TB-451e (9/04)

County of San Diego

Treating TB Infection

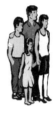

How medicine will keep you and your family healthy.

(continued)

Contact investigations should be conducted by infection control personnel in collaboration with local tuberculosis control program personnel. Community contact investigations will usually be conducted by the local health department. However, an investigation of contacts during the patient's stay or during a time that a health care worker was infectious should be performed by the facility.

Figure 4-2. Sample Resources from the CDC's TB Education and Training Resources Web Site, *continued*

Treating TB Infection

You need to read this pamphlet if:

- Your TB skin test was positive OR
- Someone close to you has contagious tuberculosis (TB).

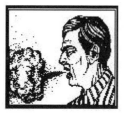

What is TB?

TB is a disease caused by a germ called Mycobacterium tuberculosis. TB can damage your lungs. Sometimes TB can occur in other parts of the body like the brain, kidneys or bones. If left untreated, TB can cripple and possibly lead to death.

How is it spread?

TB is spread when a person with contagious TB disease coughs germs into the air. Other people can then breathe these germs into their lungs and become infected.

What does a positive TB skin test mean?

A positive TB skin test means that you have TB germs in your body. This means you either have TB infection or TB disease. You need to have a chest x-ray to find out whether or not you have the disease.

TB infection is *not* the same as TB disease.

Infection means you have the TB germs but your body is fighting them. You cannot spread the germs to other people. Like most people infected with TB, you have a normal chest x-ray. However, if you are not treated, you may develop TB disease in the future.

Disease means your body was not able to fight the TB infection and you became sick with TB.

Tuberculosis usually occurs in your lungs, but can be anywhere in the body. Only people who are sick with TB in the lungs are contagious.

Why do I need medicine?

- **If your skin test was positive and your chest x-ray was normal:**

You are infected with TB. You can be treated with medication that will kill the TB germs and keep you from developing the disease. The most commonly used medication is isoniazid

or INH, although other medications may be used in some cases. Treatment with INH is usually for nine months.

- **If your skin test was negative:**

Your doctor may feel you are still at risk, because, for example you are in close contact with someone with contagious TB. Treatment may be needed to protect you. Because you can feel fine, it may be hard to take your medicine everyday. But, to get the most protection, it is important to take it regularly. There are a lot of ways to remember to take your medicine. You will want to work out your very best system, but here are two tips:

- **Take it at the same time everyday.**

 You can include taking your pill as part of your morning or evening routine such as after brushing your teeth in the morning or before bedtime.

Source: *Treating TB Infection.* San Diego County Health & Human Services Agency, Tuberculosis Control Program, San Diego, CA. Used with permission.

A contact investigation should be conducted in a health care setting when the following occurs:

- A person with tuberculosis disease has been examined at the site, and tuberculosis disease was not diagnosed and reported rapidly, resulting in a delayed application of tuberculosis infection controls.

- Environmental controls or other infection control measures have malfunctioned while a patient with tuberculosis disease was in the setting.
- A health care worker has developed tuberculosis disease and exposed other persons in the setting, either other patients or health care workers.

Figure 4-3, page 119, provides further details on how to make the decision to initiate a tuberculosis contact investigation.

When any of these situations is recognized in a health care setting, standard public health practices should be implemented to identify other patients, health care workers, and visitors who may have been exposed. This is done by doing the following:
- Notifying the local public health authority
- Interviewing the patient (known as the index case) and all individuals who might have been exposed
- Reviewing the medical records for the index case
- Determining the following possible exposure sites:
  - Where the index case lived
  - Where the index case worked
  - Places the index case visited
  - The facility at which the index case was hospitalized before being placed under airborne precautions, if the index case was hospitalized
- Determining the infectious period of the index case. (For patients with positive acid-fast bacilli [AFB] sputum smears, the infectious period should be estimated to have begun three months before the collection date of the first positive smear result or the symptom onset date, whichever is earlier. The end of the infectious period is considered to be the date the patient is placed under airborne precautions or the date of collection of the first consistently negative AFB sputum smear. For patients with negative AFB sputum smears, the infectious period can begin one month before the symptom onset date.)

Index Case
The first person with tuberculosis disease who is identified in a particular setting. This person might be an indicator of a potential public health problem and is not necessarily the source case.

Figure 4-3. Decision to Initiate a Tuberculosis Contact Investigation

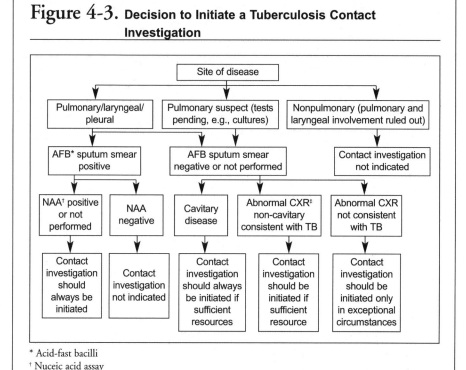

* Acid-fast bacilli
† Nuceic acid assay
‡ Chest radiograph

Source: Centers for Disease Control and Prevention: Guidelines for the investigation of contacts of persons with infectious tuberculosis. *MMWR Recomm Rep* 54, Dec. 16, 2005. http://www.cdc.gov/mmwr/preview/mmwrhtml/rr5415a1.htm (accessed Jul. 11, 2007).

When interviewing the index case patient, an interviewer needs to establish disease characteristics, onset time of illness, names of contacts, exposure locations, and current medical factors (for example, initiation of effective treatment and drug susceptibility results). Some patients might not be willing to share such extensive personal information, particularly if they have HIV or another concurrent illness, or have engaged in high-risk behavior that may have contributed to their condition. Establishing trust and consistent rapport between health care workers, public health workers, and patients, as well as educating the patient about the disease and its potential impact on his or her contacts, is critical to gaining full information and long-term cooperation during treatment. Although public health staff generally conduct these interviews, health care workers who work in the health care facility may also be called upon, particularly when the investigation pertains to a nosocomial tuberculosis infection. Good interviewing skills can be taught and learned skills improved with practice; workers assigned these tasks should be trained in interview methods and tutored on the job.

Also, be aware that the majority of tuberculosis patients in the United States today were born in other countries (*see* Chapter 1 for more detail), and their fluency in English may be insufficient for productive interviews to be conducted in English. Patients should be interviewed by persons who are fluent in their primary language or who are assisted by professional interpreters.

The exposure period should be determined, as well as whether there has been transmission to any other person with whom the index patient has had intense contact. The following need to be established:
• The intensity of the exposure for each contact based on proximity
• Overlap with the infectious period of the index case
• The duration of the exposure
• Presence or absence of infection control measures
• Infectiousness of the index case
• Performance of procedures that could increase the risk for transmission during contact (for example, sputum induction, bronchoscopy, airway suction)
• The exposed cohort of contacts for tuberculosis screening

The most intensely exposed health care workers, patients, and other contacts should be screened as quickly as possible using the tuberculin skin test (TST), and the following measures should be taken:
• Perform a symptom screen.
• Repeat the TST and symptom screen 8 to 10 weeks after the end of the exposure, if the initial TST is negative.
• Immediately evaluate the health care worker or other contact for tuberculosis disease, including a chest radiograph if the symptom screen or the initial 8- to 10-week TST result is positive.
• Provide additional medical and diagnostic evaluation for LTBI, including the determination of the extent of exposure if tuberculosis disease is excluded.

Initial Tuberculosis Training and Education
The type of initial training should vary depending on the responsibilities of the health care worker and the risk classification of the setting. For example, whereas vol-

unteers should receive basic training on how to prevent the spread of infection through cough etiquette and other such strategies, respiratory therapists should also receive training on how to keep themselves protected while inducing coughs in potential tuberculosis patients.

Educational materials on tuberculosis training are available from various sources (at no cost) in print and multimedia formats, on videotape, and online. Sidebar 4-1, pages 122–123, includes more information about some of these sources. Local or state health departments usually have additional educational materials, as well as community-specific information that can help develop a program that addresses the individual needs of your health care facility.

Suggested Components of an Initial Tuberculosis Training and Education Program

The following are the suggested components of an initial tuberculosis training and education program for health care workers, according to the CDC:

1. Clinical information
   - Basic concepts of *M. tuberculosis* transmission, pathogenesis, and diagnosis, including the difference between LTBI and tuberculosis disease and the possibility of reinfection after previous infection with *M. tuberculosis* or tuberculosis disease
   - Symptoms and signs of tuberculosis disease and the importance of a high index of suspicion for patients or health care workers with these symptoms
   - Indications for initiation of airborne precautions of inpatients with suspected or confirmed tuberculosis disease
   - Policies and indications for discontinuing airborne precautions
   - Principles of treatment for LTBI and for tuberculosis disease (indications, use, effectiveness, and potential adverse effects)
2. Epidemiology of tuberculosis
   - Epidemiology of tuberculosis in the local community, the United States, and worldwide
   - Risk factors for tuberculosis disease
3. Infection control practices to prevent and detect *M. tuberculosis* transmission in health care settings
   - Overview of the tuberculosis infection control program
   - Potential for occupational exposure to infectious tuberculosis disease in health care settings

Sidebar 4-1.
Training and Education Resources

Following are some resources that can help your organization develop a comprehensive tuberculosis education program for health care workers.

CDC's Division of Tuberculosis Elimination: http://www.cdc.gov/tb
This site includes links to just about all of the tuberculosis-related information that has been issued by the CDC, much of which is available in multiple formats, such as PDF, Microsoft® PowerPoint®, HTML, and Microsoft Word®. The 2005 guidelines, as well as treatment guidelines (which are available for download to a personal digital assistant or other handheld device), Web-based training courses, news and trends updates, frequently asked questions, and more can be found here.

TB Education & Training Resources: http://www.findtbresources.org
Developed by the CDC, this Web site provides health departments, lung associations, and providers of health care and health education the ability to upload and access materials on tuberculosis education, training, and public awareness. It also provides access to resources that offer general information about tuberculosis for patients and the general public.

Sign up at this site for the monthly e-newsletter published by the CDC's Division of Tuberculosis Elimination to learn about new resources that have been submitted to the database, locate funding resources, sign up for tuberculosis-related electronic mailing lists and digests, and more.

National Tuberculosis Curriculum Consortium: http://ntcc.ucsd.edu
This site was established under a contract from the National Heart, Lung and Blood Institute of the National Institutes of Health and is led by the University of California at San Diego School of Medicine. Although its primary goal is to help educational institutions develop curricula that effectively address tuberculosis and LTBI, it includes a great deal of information that can serve as a reference and a foundation for developing training and education programs for practicing health care workers. This includes lists of core competencies and detailed objectives for respiratory therapists, nurse practitioners, pharmacists, and other health care workers who are vital to the diagnosis and treatment of tuberculosis.

(continued)

Sidebar 4-1.
Training and Education Resources, *continued*

For example, the core competencies for pharmacists include the following:
1. Demonstrate knowledge of the following:
   a. Epidemiology of active and latent tuberculosis and risk factors for acquisition of tuberculosis
   b. Clinical syndromes associated with tuberculosis infection and differences in adult, pediatric, and HIV–infected populations
   c. Diagnostic tests for tuberculosis and interpretation of test results
   d. Treatment of tuberculosis infection
   e. Public health tuberculosis control system
   f. Available resources for updating knowledge about tuberculosis
2. Gather accurate and essential information pertinent to the diagnosis and care of patients or populations infected with tuberculosis, including medical interviews, historical records, and results of diagnostic tests and/or surveillance.
3. Formulate recommendations about pharmacologic options for patients suspected or known to have tuberculosis, incorporating knowledge of best practice and patient preferences.
4. Demonstrate interpersonal and communication skills that foster the development of effective relationships with patients and families affected by tuberculosis.
5. Apply knowledge of community and public health resources for prevention and treatment of tuberculosis to optimize health care for patients with tuberculosis and their families.

Regional Training and Medical Consultation Centers (RTMCCs):
http://www.cdc.gov/tb/rtmcc.htm
The CDC's Division of Tuberculosis Elimination funds four Tuberculosis Regional Training and Medical Consultation Centers (RTMCCs) that are regionally assigned to cover all 50 states and the U.S. territories. The primary purpose of each RTMCC is to do the following:
- Provide training and technical assistance to increase human resources development in tuberculosis programs
- Develop tuberculosis educational materials
- Provide medical consultation to tuberculosis programs and medical providers

- Principles and practices of infection control to reduce the risk for transmission of *M. tuberculosis,* including the hierarchy of tuberculosis infection control measures, written policies and procedures, monitoring, and control measures for health care workers at increased risk for exposure to *M. tuberculosis*
- Rationale for infection control measures and documentation evaluating the effect of these measures in reducing occupational tuberculosis risk exposure and *M. tuberculosis* transmission
- Reasons for testing for *M. tuberculosis* infection, importance of a positive test result for *M. tuberculosis* infection, importance of participation in a tuberculosis screening program, and importance of retaining documentation of previous test results for *M. tuberculosis* infection, chest radiograph results, and treatment for LTBI and tuberculosis disease
- Efficacy and safety of Bacille Calmette-Guérin (BCG) vaccination and principles of screening for *M. tuberculosis* infection and interpretation in BCG recipients
- Procedures for investigating an *M. tuberculosis* infection test conversion or tuberculosis disease occurring in the workplace
- Joint responsibility of health care workers and employers to ensure prompt medical evaluation after *M. tuberculosis* test conversion or development of symptoms or signs of tuberculosis disease in health care workers
- Role of health care workers in preventing transmission of *M. tuberculosis*
- Responsibility of health care workers to promptly report a diagnosis of tuberculosis disease to the setting's administration and infection control program
- Responsibility of clinicians and the infection control program to report to the state or local health department a suspected case of tuberculosis disease in a patient (including autopsy findings) or health care workers
- Responsibilities and policies of the setting, the local health department, and the state health department to ensure confidentiality for health care workers with tuberculosis disease or LTBI
- Responsibility of the setting to inform emergency medical services staff who transported a patient with suspected or confirmed tuberculosis disease
- Responsibilities and policies of the setting to ensure that a health care worker with tuberculosis disease is noninfectious before returning to duty
- Importance of completing therapy for LTBI or tuberculosis disease to protect the health care worker's health and to reduce the risk to others
- Proper implementation and monitoring of environmental controls (*see* the "Environmental Controls" section of Chapter 3, beginning on page 98)

- Training for safe collection, management, and disposal of clinical specimens
- Required Occupational Safety and Health Administration (OSHA) record keeping on health care worker test conversions for *M. tuberculosis* infection
- Record keeping and surveillance of tuberculosis cases among patients in the setting
- Proper use of (*see* "Respiratory Protection Controls," beginning on page 104) and the need to inform the infection control program of factors that might affect the efficacy of respiratory protection as required by OSHA
- Success of adherence to infection control practices in decreasing the risk for transmission of *M. tuberculosis* in health care settings

4. Tuberculosis and immunocompromising conditions
   - Relationship between infection with *M. tuberculosis* and medical conditions and treatments that can lead to impaired immunity
   - Available tests and counseling and referrals for persons with HIV infection, diabetes, and other immunocompromising conditions associated with an increased risk for progression to tuberculosis disease
   - Procedures for informing employee health or infection control personnel of medical conditions associated with immunosuppression
   - Policies on voluntary work reassignment options for immunocompromised health care workers
   - Applicable confidentiality safeguards of the health care setting, locality, and state

5. Tuberculosis and public health
   - Role of the local and state health department's tuberculosis control program in screening for LTBI and tuberculosis disease, providing treatment, conducting contact investigations and outbreak investigations, and providing education, counseling, and responses to public inquiries
   - Roles of the CDC and OSHA
   - Availability of information, advice, and counseling from community sources, including universities, local experts, and hotlines
   - Responsibility of the setting's clinicians and infection control program to promptly report to the state or local health department a case of suspected tuberculosis disease or a cluster of TST or blood assay for *M. tuberculosis* (BAMT) conversions
   - Responsibility of the setting's clinicians and infection control program to promptly report to the state or local health department a person with suspected or confirmed tuberculosis disease who leaves the setting against medical advice

Health care facilities should use this list as a foundation for developing training, making changes as appropriate depending on the health care workers' positions. In addition, the facility should keep documentation that all health care workers, including physicians, have received initial tuberculosis training relevant to their work setting and additional occupation-specific education.[4]

Follow-Up Tuberculosis Training and Education

Even in settings that are considered higher risk, health care workers in the United States do not see tuberculosis cases very often. Although this is good news for patients, it increases the likelihood that health care workers' tuberculosis-related knowledge and skills will lapse and eventually lead to errors in identification and isolation of tuberculosis patients when they are encountered.

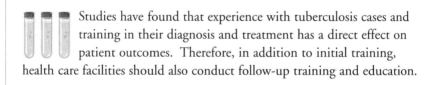 Studies have found that experience with tuberculosis cases and training in their diagnosis and treatment has a direct effect on patient outcomes. Therefore, in addition to initial training, health care facilities should also conduct follow-up training and education.

To determine when follow-up training is necessary, facilities should conduct annual evaluations to determine the number of untrained and new health care workers, the changes in the organization and services of the setting, and the availability of new tuberculosis infection control information. These factors will also help ascertain the type and level of follow-up education required.

If a potential or known exposure to *M. tuberculosis* occurs in the setting, the prevention and control measures used by the organization should include retraining health care workers on the infection control program and the procedures established to prevent the recurrence of exposure. If a potential or known exposure results in a newly recognized positive TST or BAMT result, test conversion, or diagnosis of tuberculosis disease, education should include information on the following:
1. Transmission of *M. tuberculosis*
2. Noninfectiousness of health care workers with LTBI
3. Potential infectiousness of health care workers with tuberculosis disease

In these cases, the follow-up training should be conducted as soon as possible and must be mandatory. The organization must impress upon its staff members the importance of keeping their tuberculosis knowledge up-to-date, particularly in a time of potential and actual exposures.

Health care workers in settings with a risk classification of *potential ongoing transmission* should receive additional training and education on (1) symptoms and signs of tuberculosis disease, (2) *M. tuberculosis* transmission, (3) infection control policies, (4) importance of tuberculosis screening for health care workers, and (5) responsibilities of employers and employees regarding *M. tuberculosis* infection test conversion and diagnosis of tuberculosis disease.

In addition, OSHA requires that health care workers who use respiratory devices receive annual respiratory protection training. More information on respiratory protection can be found in Chapter 3.

References

1. Chalco K.: Nurses as providers of emotional support to patients with MDR-TB. *Int Nurs Rev* 53:253–60, Dec. 2006.
2. Clark P.M.: Effect of pharmacist-led patient education on adherence to tuberculosis treatment. *Am J Health Syst Pharm* 64:497–506, Mar. 1, 2007.
3. Kellerman S.E.: APIC and CDC survey of *Mycobacterium tuberculosis* isolation and control practices in hospitals caring for children. Part 2: Environmental and administrative controls. *Am J Infect Control* 26:483–487, 1998.
4. Munoz F.: Tuberculosis among adult visitors of children with suspected tuberculosis and employees at a children's hospital. *Infect Control Hosp Epidemiol* 23:568–572, 2002.

Chapter 5

International Implications

Although tuberculosis infections in the United States are at a current all-time low, rates in developing countries continue to rise. The global incidence rate continues to grow by 1% each year: There are nine million new tuberculosis cases each year and two million tuberculosis deaths. In addition, about one third of the world's population has a latent tuberculosis infection (LTBI) that could develop into tuberculosis disease in years to come.[1]

Historically, tuberculosis has been primarily a disease of poverty, as poverty is often associated with overcrowding, poor ventilation, malnutrition, and other conditions that result in greater transmission of the disease. Today, poverty is also associated with a high incidence of other infectious diseases, such as HIV/AIDS, so that many patients suffer from another serious illness in addition to tuberculosis. Thus, treatment of tuberculosis is growing increasingly difficult. Concurrent HIV and tuberculosis infections are particularly problematic in South Africa, where virulent strains resistant to all standard drugs killed 52 of 53 patients in 2005 and 2006.[2]

In response to these issues, in 2000, the World Health Organization (WHO) founded the Stop TB Partnership to eliminate tuberculosis as a public health problem and ultimately to realize a world free of the disease. The partnership is a network of more than 500 international organizations, countries, donors from the public and private sectors, and nongovernmental and governmental organizations that have expressed an interest in working together to achieve this goal.

Shortly after its formation, the partnership created *The Global Plan to Stop TB 2001–2005,* which provided an agenda to rally new key partners, push forward research and development, and have a rapid impact on tuberculosis in the areas suffering most from the epidemic. This plan differed from previous tuberculosis-related plans in that instead of a vertical approach, which had not met with great success in the past,[3] it took a more integrated approach, based on advocacy and involving communities and a variety of for-profit and not-for-profit organizations in the effort.

The new plan design was largely successful: The number of patients treated in directly observed therapy and directly observed therapy, short course (DOTS) programs more than doubled over five years, from two million in 2000 to more than four million in 2004. As a result, several high-burden countries, such as India and China, are close to reaching the target of 70% case detection. There has also been significant progress in research and development, with a number of new diagnostics, drugs, and vaccines in the pipeline.

Yet there is still much work to be done, particularly in Africa and Southeast Asia (*see* Table 5-1, page 131). This is why the Stop TB Partnership has issued *The Global Plan to Stop TB 2006–2015.*

Implications of the WHO's *The Global Plan to Stop TB 2006–2015*

As part of the Stop TB Strategy outlined in the plan, the Stop TB Partnership plans to take the following steps:

1. Pursue quality DOTS expansion and enhancement, improving case-finding and cure through an effective patient-centered approach to reach all patients, particularly the poor.
2. Address tuberculosis/HIV, multidrug-resistant tuberculosis (MDR-TB), and other challenges by scaling up tuberculosis/HIV joint activities, DOTS-Plus, and other relevant approaches.
3. Contribute to health system strengthening by collaborating with other health programs and general services, for example, in mobilizing the necessary human and financial resources for implementation and impact evaluation, and in sharing and applying achievements of tuberculosis control.
4. Involve all care providers—public, nongovernmental, and private—by scaling up approaches based on a public-private mix (PPM), to ensure adherence to the International Standards of TB Care (which will be addressed later in this chapter).
5. Engage people with tuberculosis and affected communities to demand and contribute to effective care. This will involve scaling up community tuberculosis care; creating demand through context-specific advocacy, communication, and social mobilization; and supporting development of a patient's charter for the tuberculosis community.

Table 5-1. Estimated Tuberculosis Incidence, Prevalence, and Mortality—2005

WHO Region	Incidence*					Prevalence*		Mortality	
	All Forms		Smear-Positive[†]						
	Number (thousands)	Per 100,000 Pop[‡]	Number (Thousands)	Per 100,000 Pop[‡]		Number (Thousands)	Per 100,000 Pop[‡]	Number (Thousands)	Per 100,000 Pop[‡]
	(% of Global Total)								
Africa	2,529 (29)	343	1,088	147		3,773	511	544	74
The Americas	352 (4)	39	157	18		448	50	49	5.5
Eastern Mediterranean	565 (6)	104	253	47		881	163	112	21
Europe	445 (5)	50	199	23		525	60	66	7.4
Southeast Asia	2,993 (34)	181	1,339	81		4,809	290	512	31
Western Pacific	1,927 (22)	110	866	49		3,616	206	295	17
Global	**8,811 (100)**	**136**	**3,902**	**60**		**14,052**	**217**	**1,578**	**24**

* Incidence, New cases arising in given period; Prevalence, the number of cases that exist in the population at a given point in time.
†Smear-positive cases are those confirmed by smear microscopy, and are the most infectious cases.
‡"Pop" indicates population.

Source: World Health Organization: *Tuberculosis: Infection and Transmission.* Fact sheet no. 104, Mar. 2007. http://www.who.int/mediacentre/factsheets/fs104/en/index.html (accessed Jul. 11, 2007).

6. Enable and promote research for the development of new drugs, diagnostics, and vaccines. Research will also be needed to improve program performance.

If the plan is fully implemented, the partnership believes it will achieve the following:

- Implementation of the Stop TB Strategy will expand equitable access to quality tuberculosis diagnosis and treatment.
- Over the 10 years of this plan, about 50 million people will be treated for tuberculosis under the Stop TB Strategy, including about 800,000 patients with MDR-TB, and about 3 million patients who have both tuberculosis and HIV will be enrolled on antiretroviral therapy (in line with the Joint United Nations Programme on HIV/AIDS plans for universal access).
- Some 14 million lives will be saved from 2006 to 2015.
- The first new tuberculosis drug in 40 years will be introduced in 2010, with a new short tuberculosis regimen (one to two months) shortly after 2015.
- By 2010, diagnostic tests at the point of care will allow rapid, sensitive, and inexpensive detection of active tuberculosis. By 2012, a diagnostic toolbox will accurately identify people with LTBI and those at high risk of progression to disease.
- By 2015, a new, safe, effective, and affordable vaccine will be available with potential for a significant impact on tuberculosis control in later years.

Although implementation of the plan is underway, the WHO and the partnership are still in the process of obtaining full funding for the programs. Full funding (U.S. $56 billion) would result in the following:

- Global achievement of the United Nation's Millennium Development Goal 6, Target 8: to have halted by 2015, and begun to reverse, the incidence of malaria and other major diseases, including tuberculosis
- Global achievement of the partnership's 2015 targets to halve prevalence and death rates from the 1990 baseline (although achievement of the 2015 targets will most likely be later than 2015 in Eastern Europe and even later in Africa because of the particular challenges posed by MDR-TB and HIV, respectively)
- Enormous progress in all regions over the period of the plan from 2006 to 2015, with prevalence and death rates halved, or almost halved

The Impact of DOTS

DOTS has proven to be one of the most effective treatment strategies because it includes not only direct observation to ensure that the patient is taking the medication properly, but also some additional elements. These additional elements include the following[4]:

1. *Political Commitment with Increased and Sustained Financing*
   Political commitment should be backed up by legislation to ensure that the nation's leadership continues to support the program.
2. *Case Detection Through Quality-Assured Bacteriology*
   This requires a network of well-equipped laboratories with well-trained staff, as well as improved testing techniques.
3. *Standardized Treatment with Supervision and Patient Support*
   DOTS is effective only with supervision; factors that may make patients interrupt or stop treatment must be identified and addressed. Access to care must also be adequate.
4. *An Effective Drug Supply and Management System*
   An uninterrupted and sustained supply of quality-assured antituberculosis drugs is fundamental to tuberculosis control. For this purpose, an effective drug supply and management system is essential.
5. *Monitoring and Evaluation System, and Impact Measurement*
   When compiled and analysed, data from a DOTS program can be used at the facility level to monitor treatment outcomes, at the district level to identify local problems as they arise, at the provincial or national level to ensure consistently high-quality tuberculosis control across geographical areas, and nationally and internationally to evaluate the performance of each country.[8]

While DOTS has proven to be an effective tuberculosis control strategy, there are still some challenges to implementing and sustaining such programs for the long term. These include failures of governmental bodies to develop the appropriate health systems and a lack of community support. To help address these concerns, in 2002, WHO's Stop TB department published *An Expanded DOTS Framework for Effective Tuberculosis Control.* This document emphasizes the following:

- Public health services need to enhance their capacity to sustain and expand DOTS implementation without compromising the quality of case detection and treatment.
- Community involvement in tuberculosis care and a patient-centered approach need emphasis and promotion to improve both access to and utilization of health services.
- Collaboration and synergy among the public, private, and voluntary sectors are essential to ensure accessible and quality-assured tuberculosis diagnosis and treatment.
- The increasing impact of HIV on the incidence of tuberculosis, particularly in sub-Saharan Africa, calls for new partnerships and approaches.

- A surge in drug-resistant forms of tuberculosis in the former Soviet Union and several other parts of the world requires effective implementation of the DOTS strategy to prevent occurrence of new MDR-TB cases, as well as measures to cure existing cases.
- Sustaining DOTS programs will require that they be integrated into primary health care and adapted to ongoing reforms within health sectors worldwide.

This expanded strategy lays equal emphasis on the technical, managerial, social, and political dimensions of DOTS. In addition, it reinforces the WHO's stance that access to tuberculosis care is a human right and that tuberculosis control is a social good with large benefits to society.[5]

The Effects of Concurring MDR-TB and Extremely Drug-Resistant Tuberculosis

Drug-resistant strains of tuberculosis can arise as a result of improper treatment regimens or failure to ensure that patients complete the whole course of treatment. One patient with drug-resistant tuberculosis can then transmit that strain of the disease to another person, just as with any other form of pulmonary tuberculosis.

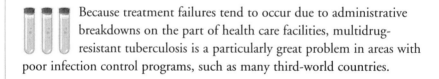 Because treatment failures tend to occur due to administrative breakdowns on the part of health care facilities, multidrug-resistant tuberculosis is a particularly great problem in areas with poor infection control programs, such as many third-world countries.

When a patient with MDR-TB (resistant to first-line treatment drugs) or extremely drug-resistant tuberculosis (XDR-TB; resistant to first-line drugs and some second-line drugs) also suffers from another serious illness, such as HIV, each condition exacerbates the other, making it extremely difficult to treat the patient.

Of additional concern is the recent discovery of tuberculosis strains that are resistant to all drug therapies. A recent study of patients with drug-resistant tuberculosis in Italy and Germany found two cases that were resistant to all first- and second-line medications.[6]

Strategies for preventing the transmission of drug-resistant tuberculosis are the same as for drug-susceptible tuberculosis. However, health care facilities can help prevent the development of further strains of the disease by ensuring that health care workers are properly trained on treatment of tuberculosis and that patients are educated on the importance of continuing treatment. (For more information on drug-resistant tuberculosis, *see* Chapter 1.)

Developments in Diagnostics, Pharmaceuticals, and Vaccines

Many experts feel that the keys to controlling tuberculosis worldwide will be diagnostic testing that is less complicated and takes less time, drug therapies that are less costly and complex and do not require such long treatment periods, and more effective vaccines. For example, quicker diagnostic procedures will allow health care workers to begin providing appropriate treatment and isolation sooner (if necessary), thus decreasing the opportunities for that patient to transmit the disease to others. In addition, a treatment that takes a few days rather than a few months, or just one medication instead of four, will be much easier for health care facilities to monitor, particularly in countries with less-established health care and technology infrastructures. Such treatments will also be less of a drain on health care facilities' staff time and financial resources (*see* Sidebar 5-1, page 136, for an alternative view of this issue).

The Global Alliance for TB Drug Development

Also known as the TB Alliance, the Global Alliance for TB Drug Development is one organization that is looking to solve this portion of the global tuberculosis crisis. This not-for-profit, product development partnership of representatives from academia, industry, major agencies, nongovernmental organizations, and donors is working to accelerate the discovery and development of new tuberculosis drugs that will shorten treatment, be effective against drug-susceptible and drug-resistant strains, be compatible with antiretroviral therapies for tuberculosis patients who also have HIV, and improve treatment of LTBI.

The TB Alliance is committed not only to developing these new drugs, but also to ensuring that approved new regimens are affordable, adopted, and available to those who need them. Recognizing that new, faster, and better tuberculosis drugs will be effective only if they are affordable and available, the TB Alliance and its partners are working with global, regional, and national stakeholders to ensure regulatory approval, adoption by tuberculosis programs, and widespread availability of new drug regimens.

Sidebar 5-1.
Do We Already Have a Quicker Cure?

At a 2007 meeting of the International Consortium for Trials of Chemotherapeutic Agents in Tuberculosis, some researchers argued that development of
new drug therapies takes much too long, and to truly have an impact on controlling tuberculosis, the scientific community should focus on new uses of
existing drugs. Some believe that higher doses of current tuberculosis drugs,
such as rifampicin, will allow for a shorter treatment time and might overcome
some drug resistance; others say that we should look to drugs used to treat other
illnesses, such as moxifloxacin, an antibiotic used for suchbacterial infections as
conjunctivitis.

Source: Hargreaves S.: Existing tuberculosis drugs may hold key to shorter treatment. *Lancet Infect Dis* 7:309, 2007.

Currently, the TB Alliance has two drugs in clinical trials and many more in the
research and development process. As new treatments are developed, the TB Alliance
seeks to reduce the treatment time for tuberculosis to two months; in the long term,
the organization would like to bring that time down to two weeks.

The Need to Strengthen Health Care Systems and Processes

If any tuberculosis control program is to succeed, a country must have the infrastructure to provide the necessary support, funding, and staffing. The Pan American
Health Organization (PAHO) has developed a plan that was designed with the
Americas in mind but could be adapted to other regions as well. *The Regional Plan
for Tuberculosis Control, 2006–2015* includes the following strategies[7]:

1. Expand and/or strengthen the DOTS strategy, ensuring its quality application.
2. Implement and/or strengthen the following:
   - Tuberculosis and HIV/AIDS interprogram collaborative activities
   - MDR-TB prevention and control activities
   - Community strategies for neglected populations (for example, indigenous pop-
     ulations, prisoners, periurban neglected populations)

3. Strengthen the health system, emphasizing primary care, a comprehensive approach to respiratory diseases (Practical Approach to Lung Health [PAL] Strategy), the laboratory network, and the development of tuberculosis human resource policies.
4. Improve the population's access to tuberculosis diagnosis and treatment through the inclusion of all health care providers, both public and private.
5. Empower affected persons and the community, and implement advocacy, communications, and social mobilization (ACSM).
6. Include operations, clinical, and epidemiological research in national tuberculosis control program plans.

The plan also includes country-specific and region-specific action steps to be taken to implement each of these strategies. The followins sections discuss some of the country-specific activities the PAHO recommends.

Expand/Strengthen the DOTS Strategy to Ensure Quality Application

The five steps detailed by the WHO as part of the expansion of the DOTS efforts make up the first part of this strategy. In addition, the PAHO recommends the following steps for all countries, regardless of tuberculosis incidence:

- Obtain and/or maintain ongoing political commitment at different levels through advocacy activities involving different sectors of society.
- Integrate technical, financial, and social partners into control activities through the formation of interagency Stop TB committees—including partners who traditionally work in tuberculosis, as well as new ones such as scientific societies, specialist physicians, networks of DOTS nursing and allied health professionals, community organizations, associations of affected persons, and private service institutions—to successfully implement long-term, sustainable, quality DOTS.
- Strengthen the tuberculosis epidemiological surveillance system and integrate it into the countries' national epidemiological surveillance systems.
- Promote, technically support, and evaluate border, binational, or multinational cooperation agreements for tuberculosis management.
- Prepare and implement projects to increase the flow of economic resources.

Implement/Strengthen Community Activities and Strategies

Tuberculosis and HIV/AIDS Interprogram Collaborative Activities

The PAHO recommends that action steps in this area be grouped according to a country's tuberculosis and HIV incidence rates to ensure that immediate and long-term needs of these areas are addressed.

For countries with generalized HIV epidemic, the PAHO suggests the following:
- Establishing interprogram collaboration mechanisms aimed at the following:
  - Forming working groups and expert committees on tuberculosis/HIV management
  - Reviewing and/or updating national tuberculosis program (NTP) technical standards, including management of tuberculosis/HIV coinfection
  - Establishing and/or strengthening the epidemiological surveillance system through data collection on the routine care of tuberculosis patients (HIV counseling and voluntary testing in every tuberculosis case)
- Decreasing the tuberculosis burden in patients living with HIV by doing the following:
  - Intensifying case-finding for tuberculosis in people living with HIV or AIDS
  - Introducing preventive treatment with isoniazid
- Decreasing the HIV burden in tuberculosis patients by doing the following:
  - Providing counseling and voluntary HIV testing for tuberculosis patients
  - Promoting HIV prevention among tuberculosis patients
  - Introducing prevention of opportunistic infections in coinfected people
  - Ensuring comprehensive care of people living with HIV or AIDS
  - Introducing and/or strengthening antiretroviral therapy

In countries with concentrated or incipient HIV epidemic, the PAHO recommends the following:
- Establishing interprogram collaboration mechanisms by doing the following:
  - Forming working groups and expert committees on tuberculosis/HIV management
  - Reviewing and/or updating NTP technical standards, including management of tuberculosis/HIV coinfection
  - Decreasing the burden of tuberculosis in people living with HIV/AIDS with specific actions targeting risk groups (men who have sex with men, drug users, sex workers, and confined populations) and in areas in which the prevalence in pregnant women is higher than the national average
- Establishing and/or strengthening the epidemiological surveillance system, based on the following:
  - Data collection on the routine care of tuberculosis patients (HIV counseling and voluntary testing in every tuberculosis case)
  - Establishment of sentinel surveillance and/or periodic prevalence surveys in countries that cannot conduct routine surveillance

MDR-TB Prevention and Control Activities
In accordance with WHO directives, the PAHO has made the following recommendations:
- Strengthening of the DOTS strategy
- Preparation, implementation, and expansion of MDR-TB management projects in areas where the DOTS strategy is being used with good results
- Identification and correction of the causes of multidrug resistance in the countries by the following:
  - Guaranteeing drug quality
  - Strengthening the laboratories and drug quality control procedures
  - Promoting mechanisms that limit the indiscriminate sale of first- and second-line drugs
  - Promoting the use of fixed-dose drug combinations
  - Using the supply mechanism for second-line drugs and the technical support of the Tropical Disease Foundation's Green Light Committee
- Strengthening of the MDR-TB surveillance system by doing the following:
  - Systematically monitoring drug resistance in all cases of Category 1 treatment failure
  - Conducting national studies of primary and secondary resistance to evaluate patterns of MDR-TB

Community Strategies for Neglected Populations
As this is a regional issue, the PAHO did not make any country-specific recommendations in this area, but rather urged countries to identify those regions within their borders that could use the following support:
- Advise on the preparation of intervention plans to assist the countries in addressing tuberculosis in poor populations.
- Encourage the countries and NTPs to commit to adopting and developing policies and strategies aimed at addressing the problems in these population groups.
- Facilitate regional meetings with country experts in order to share experiences, set criteria for prioritizing populations, and establish lines of intervention, emphasizing prisoners, indigenous populations, and marginal populations in large cities.
- Contribute to the development of materials for training, information, and guidelines.
- Facilitate strategic partnerships for the mobilization of resources and establish coordination with the PAHO's Health Services Unit.

Strengthen the Health System

To strengthen the laboratory network, the PAHO recommends the following activities:

- Coordinate technical cooperation with the supranational reference laboratories (SRLs) and collaborating centers (CCs).
- Guarantee the efficient flow of information between the NTP and the national laboratory network, and between the laboratory network's national reference laboratory and the SRLs and CCs.
- Include the people responsible for the tuberculosis laboratory network in NTP management teams.
- Conduct annual situational diagnoses, establish medium-term efficiency goals, and monitor and evaluate the performance of the tuberculosis laboratory network.
- Identify a line in the NTP budget that includes the necessary resources for the operation of the laboratory network and the achievement of program goals.
- Promote the implementation of programs aimed at achieving quality assurance in sputum-smear microscopy, culture, and sensitivity tests of first-line drugs.
- Streamline the procedures (including administrative procedures) that affect the time between requests for sputum-smear microscopy and tests of sensitivity to first-line drugs and the use of the results.
- Promote the establishment of infrastructure, equipment, and laboratory practices that follow international biosafety recommendations.
- Institute a program for the calibration, maintenance, and repair of laboratory equipment.
- Include or update the quality control and biosafety chapters in the NTP's technical standards.
- Design and implement a training program to maintain the technical competencies of the human resources in the tuberculosis laboratory network, in coordination with the NTP and based on the results of the situational diagnosis.
- Increase and optimize the use of culture for diagnosis and treatment assessment.
- Involve the tuberculosis laboratory network in the operations research planned by the NTP.
- Design, implement, and/or share operations, national, international, and/or multicenter studies to generate evidence that improves the services provided by the laboratory networks.

Other activities are also recommended based on the individual situations in each country.

Sputum

Mucus containing secretions coughed up from inside the lungs. Tests of sputum (for example, smear and culture) can confirm pulmonary tuberculosis disease. Sputum is different from saliva or nasal secretions, which are unsatisfactory specimens for detecting tuberculosis disease. However, specimens suspected to be inadequate should still be processed because positive culture results can still be obtained and might be the only bacteriologic indication of disease.

PAL Health Strategy

The PAL was developed to help health care facilities manage patients who present with respiratory symptoms at health services in areas with DOTS coverage. It offers standardized interventions to provide an appropriate cost-effective response for areas in which there is a high demand for services to treat respiratory symptoms in patients over the age of 5. The PAL recommends the following:

- In countries that have initiated the PAL, activities should be periodically monitored and evaluated, and preparations should be made for expansion of the strategy.
- In countries with low and medium estimated tuberculosis incidence and more than 90% of the population covered by DOTS, but which have not yet implemented the PAL, the PAHO recommends that the PAL strategy be put into place.
- In countries with low and medium estimated tuberculosis incidence and more than 90% of the population covered by DOTS, but which have not yet implemented the PAL, the PAHO recommends that the PAL be implemented after the plan for DOTS quality consolidation.
- In countries with high estimated tuberculosis incidence and less than 75% of the population covered by DOTS, officials should implement the PAL after successfully finalizing quality DOTS expansion and preparing a plan for its support and consolidation.

Support for Tuberculosis Human Resources Management Policies and Knowledge Dissemination

DOTS is effective largely because of the direct involvement of health care workers in the treatment process. However, this also makes DOTS difficult to implement because of the staff time involved. To address this issue, the PAHO recommends the following:

- Identify the entities in the country that can support the NTP in human resources management for the program.
- Evaluate the current status of human resources available for DOTS strategy implementation, taking into account numbers, distribution, capacity, and motivation.
- Increase monitoring, supervision, and evaluation activities of an educational rather than an enforcement nature.
- Create, implement, and strengthen methodologies that identify performance deficiencies related to the lack of skills and that make it possible to plan educational actions (formal or on-the-job training).
- Develop or improve training plans to guarantee that new tuberculosis control staff members participate in orientation and training programs as soon as they start a new position.
- Implement or improve existing tuberculosis control training programs.
- Form partnerships with universities, scientific associations, and other institutions that train health human resources to foster multidisciplinary centers of excellence that provide comprehensive support for tuberculosis control policies and activities in the country.
- Analyze and review basic training programs for physicians, nurses, laboratory professionals, and other health care professionals who participate in the implementation or expansion of the DOTS strategy, and promote their professional development.
- Coordinate training activities with other tuberculosis-related programs, such as the national HIV/AIDS program.
- Promote the appointment of a national-level official who serves as the focal point for the issue of tuberculosis human resources.
- Implement a monitoring system for tuberculosis human resources that includes the utilization of personnel databases.

Improve the Population's Access to Tuberculosis Diagnosis and Treatment

A framework that includes both private and public health care providers can create a more integrated system that ensures that patients with tuberculosis symptoms get the appropriate treatment as quickly as possible. To implement such a framework, the following should occur:

- Conduct situation studies that permit the following:
  - Identification and preparation of a list of suppliers existing in the country or region where the strategy is being implemented
  - Determination of how many and which of these suppliers have a relationship with the NTP and implement tuberculosis control activities

– Definition of the current or potential contribution of each of them to tuberculosis control
– Identification of those interventions that optimize their contribution
- Identify and generate national resources. Prepare the following plan for the implementation of PPM (public-private mix) DOTS in accordance with data contributed by the situation study:
  – Designate a person in charge of PPM in the NTP.
  – Create a PPM DOTS working group (NTP and representatives of different relevant suppliers).
  – Prepare an operations plan for implementation.
  – Identify economic resources for essential activities (for example, advocacy, training, supervision and monitoring, incentives).
- Prepare practical operations guidelines or adapt the WHO PPM DOTS guidelines. Identify working tools (letters of agreement, contracts, commitments, and instruments for records and information).

Empower Affected Persons and the Community and Implement ACSM

Empowerment strategies include the following:
- Promoting a sense of responsibility and ownership at the grassroots level
- Participatory assessments to analyze obstacles to detecting people with tuberculosis and suggesting actions to overcome them
- Supporting social networks that contribute to early detection
- Identifying social mechanisms and strategies for encouraging patients to complete their treatment
- Educational activities at the grassroots level (for example, group talks, experience sharing, presentations by people who are directly affected) to reduce the stigma of tuberculosis and of affected persons, and to address the lack of information on rights and responsibilities and the low perception of risk
- Joint efforts with health care workers to carry out support activities in DOTS centers (for example, administration of drugs, monitoring, home visits)
- Identifying grassroots-level institutional resources (for example, among civil society and the private sector) to support activities
- Promoting mechanisms for working with families to understand and mitigate the impact of tuberculosis through care and counseling
- Supporting the activities and sustainability of patients' organizations and their involvement in educational tasks, participating in sharing local experiences at national and international forums, designing and running activities, and fundraising

Strategies for implementing ACSM include the following:

- Identifying people and organizations specializing in communications and establishing joint coordination, planning, and execution of activities
- Preparing and implementing a tuberculosis communication strategy in accordance with the priorities of each NTP and based on baseline assessment results
- Involving patients and patient groups in community assessments and educational activities, in presentations with partners and authorities, and in designing and conducting communications campaigns
- Supporting the formation of associations of people affected by tuberculosis and offering training on different aspects of tuberculosis control
- Holding working meetings with health care workers and affected persons to identify ways to collaborate
- Promoting the establishment of national coalitions to discuss and support tuberculosis control activities

Include Operations, Clinical, and Epidemiological Research in National Tuberculosis Control Program Plans

These types of research are vital to continually improving national tuberculosis programs by providing administrative and clinical data that can help ensure that the NTP is serving as many patients as possible. The following are some steps a country can take:

- Identifying operations research topics, in accordance with the analysis of surveillance data and the implementation plans of new initiatives, and preparing, implementing, and disseminating research protocols
- Identifying epidemiological studies that can measure the impact of control measures and measure fulfillment of the millennium development goals targets, as well as the impact of major projects (for example, Global Fund to Fight AIDS, Tuberculosis, and Malaria)
- Participating in multicenter clinical studies, depending on the NTP's level of development
- Conducting social and/or socioanthropological studies to identify strategies that modify undesirable behavior (regarding tuberculosis control) in the population
- Establishing connections between the NTP and national organizations that conduct and finance scientific and technological research in order to stimulate activity among the latter on topics of interest in tuberculosis control
- Actively intervening in the mobilization of national or international funds to finance research
- Disseminating research findings at national and international levels

Tuberculosis and Air Travel

A recent case of an American who traveled internationally on a commercial airline knowing that he had tuberculosis provoked some serious discussions about how countries can protect their borders from infectious diseases—or whether they can really do so at all. (Sidebar 5-2, page 146, provides a more detailed account of that incident.)

Air quality on most commercial aircraft is quite high, and under normal conditions, cabin air is cleaner than the air in most buildings. Therefore, on short flights, there is minimal risk of disease transmission. On flights of eight hours or more, however, the extended time confined in the aircraft cabin may involve an increased risk of transmission of *Mycobacterium tuberculosis.*

To prevent the possibility of exposure to tuberculosis on airplanes, the Centers for Disease Control and Prevention (CDC) and the WHO recommend that people with infectious tuberculosis travel by private transportation (that is, not by commercial airplanes or other commercial carriers), if they must travel. This can be difficult to enforce, however, as some tuberculosis patients do not appear to be sick. The CDC and the WHO have issued guidelines for notifying passengers who might have been exposed to tuberculosis aboard airplanes in the publication *Tuberculosis and Air Travel: Guidelines for Prevention and Control.*

Exposure

A situation in which persons (for example, health care workers, visitors, inmates) have been exposed to a person with suspected or confirmed infectious tuberculosis disease (or to air containing *M. tuberculosis*) without the benefit of effective infection control measures.

The following sections discuss additional recommendations from that publication.

For Passengers and Air Crew

1. People with infectious tuberculosis must postpone long-distance travel (total flight exceeding eight hours) until they become noninfectious (completion of at least two weeks of adequate treatment) and according to the recommendations of their physicians.
2. People with MDR-TB must postpone any air travel until advised by their physicians that they are no longer infectious (for example, culture-negative).

Sidebar 5-2.
Tuberculosis Patient's Trip Raises Questions About Tuberculosis Transmission During Travel

In the spring of 2007, one tuberculosis patient's sojourn from the United States to Europe and Canada raised some important questions about a nation's ability and responsibility to restrict travel for infectious individuals. It also elicited concerns about the U.S. health system's readiness to handle a serious medical crisis or bioterrorism attack.

This incident has raised questions about whether any country can truly defend its borders against infectious diseases. To assist in this process, the CDC is currently working to increase its number of quarantine officers. In 1953 the CDC had 600 quarantine officers, but as the incidence of diseases such as smallpox and polio was significantly reduced, so was the number of quarantine officers. In 2004 there were just 70, but as of July 2007 there were 83.

Source: Altman L.K.: Agent at border, aware, let in man with TB. *New York Times,* Jun. 1, 2007.

For Physicians

3. Physicians should inform all infectious tuberculosis patients that they must not travel by air on a flight exceeding eight hours until they have completed at least two weeks of adequate treatment.

4. Physicians should inform all MDR-TB patients that they must not travel by air—under any circumstances or on a flight of any duration—until they are proven to be culture-negative.

5. Physicians should advise tuberculosis patients who undertake unavoidable air travel of short duration (less than eight hours) to wear a surgical mask when possible or to cover the nose and mouth when speaking or coughing at all times during the flight. (This recommendation is applied only on a case-by-case basis and subject to prior agreement of the airline[s] involved and the public health authorities at departure and arrival.)

6. Physicians should inform the relevant health authority when they are aware of an infectious tuberculosis patient's intention to travel against medical advice.

Mask
A device worn over the nose and mouth of a person with suspected or confirmed infectious tuberculosis disease to prevent infectious particles from being released into room air.

7. Physicians should immediately inform the relevant health authority when an infectious tuberculosis patient has a recent history of air travel (for example, within three months).

For Public Health Authorities

8. Public health authorities who are aware that a person with infectious tuberculosis is planning to travel with a commercial carrier on a flight whose total duration could potentially exceed eight hours should inform the concerned airline.
9. Health authorities should promptly contact the airline when an infectious tuberculosis patient is known to have traveled on a commercial flight of at least eight hours' duration (including ground delay time) within the preceding three months.
10. Health authorities should promptly contact potentially exposed passengers and crew and advise them to seek medical evaluation.
11. Public health authorities should establish country-specific policies and provide guidance to airlines on the prevention of risks due to infectious diseases.

For Airline Companies

12. Airline companies should deny boarding to any person who is known to have infectious tuberculosis and is intending to travel on a flight whose total duration is likely to be at least eight hours.
13. Airline companies should minimize ground delays to less than 30 minutes if the ventilation system is not in operation.
14. Airline companies should ensure that high efficiency particulate air filters on all aircraft are changed regularly according to the recommendations of the filter manufacturer.
15. Airline companies should ensure that cabin crews receive adequate training on potential exposure to infectious diseases, in first aid, and in using universal precautions when there may be exposure to body fluids.
16. Airline companies should ensure that there are adequate emergency medical supplies aboard all aircraft (including gloves, surgical masks, and biohazard disposal bags).

17. Airline companies should cooperate with health authorities in providing all contact information needed by them and facilitate contact tracing of passengers and/or crew.

Global "Hot Spots" for Tuberculosis

As seen in Table 5-1 at the beginning of this chapter, some areas of the world have much higher rates of tuberculosis than others. This is particularly true for third-world countries, where poverty, poor access to health care, and concurrently high rates of HIV create an environment in which tuberculosis can be easily transmitted and often goes untreated. The following sections discuss the tuberculosis situation in some of these areas of the world.

China and Southeast Asia

Although these areas have some of the highest incidence of tuberculosis in the world, they also have some of the highest rates of improvement since 2005 and are expected to continue improving for the duration of the 2006–2015 WHO plan.

One of the reasons for China's significant improvement is a political commitment to tuberculosis control. The government has made a clear decision to meet global targets for diagnosis and has provided the funding to do so. As a result, the country has nearly 100% DOTS coverage, leading to case detection rates of more than 70% and treatment success of more than 85%.[9]

The challenge now is to maintain that level of support and ensure that health care facilities have the staff and resources they need to continue their progress. China must also work to slow the growth of MDR-TB strains in that country; it is estimated that more than 30% of the world's MDR-TB cases are in China.

Southeast Asia, which includes a number of high-burden countries, has achieved 100% DOTS coverage. Case detection has gone from just 18% in 2000 to 45% in 2003, and was estimated to be about 65% in 2005. The treatment rate has exceeded the 2005 target of 85%. These improvements have been possible because of improved infrastructure, a reliable drug supply, increased staffing, improved laboratory services, and intensified training and supervision.

However, an estimated 35% of cases are still not being reached through existing DOTS services; southeast Asian countries should step up efforts to link all health care providers to the DOTS program. Also, this region has been among the hardest hit by the HIV epidemic: More than six million people were believed to be living with the virus as of December 2004. In addition, it is difficult to assess the MDR-TB prevalence in this region because of a lack of data from some countries.

Sub-Saharan Africa

Tuberculosis control in this region faces some serious challenges, not the least of which is the prevalence of HIV. Treatment success rates in Africa are just over 70%— far below the target rate of 85%—and that figure has been relatively unchanged since 1998. This rate is partly due to the high rates of death among people with HIV or AIDS, as well as high rates of treatment interruption.

The concurrence of HIV and tuberculosis is changing the usual demographics of tuberculosis in Africa. In general, more men than women get tuberculosis; in Russia in 2004, for example, 71% of tuberculosis patients were male and 29% were female. (These results, which are typical, are believed to be due to epidemiological differences between the sexes.) However, in areas of sub-Saharan Africa where HIV is prevalent, more women than men have HIV—and therefore, more women have tuberculosis as well.

In addition, Africa is seeing increasing rates of XDR-TB. A recent epidemic in South Africa has induced the WHO to send a permanent staff member to that country to advise authorities struggling with the outbreak.[10]

Ministers of Health from 46 member states of the Africa region unanimously declared tuberculosis an emergency in the region in August 2005. This declaration urged African countries to develop and implement, with immediate effect, emergency strategies and plans to keep the tuberculosis epidemic from worsening. This declaration of emergency will be crucial in accelerating the implementation of priority activities and in garnering the necessary commitments from all stakeholders, both nationally and internationally. Steps that African countries will need to implement include improving DOTS coverage, fostering collaboration between HIV– and tuberculosis-related organizations and health care facilities, and further decentralizing services so that individuals in rural areas have the necessary access to health care.

Cost factors are also associated with case-detection rates of tuberculosis in the region. Because of the profound connection between poverty and tuberculosis, the economic burden of diagnosis in underdeveloped countries must be reduced. In Malawi-Lilongwe, tuberculosis services are in theory universally available, as they are accessible within six kilometers and provided free of charge, but the actual cost of diagnosis for the patient is high, averaging U.S. $29, or 51 days of income. The cost to the poor in this region is staggering: 244% of their total monthly income, which rises to 574% when essential expenditures on food are excluded.

This cost reflects the burden on patients who have access to tuberculosis diagnosis, but is also likely to be a barrier for people with tuberculosis, particularly the poor, who do not have access to care. This implies that scaling up tuberculosis services to reach the poor will need to go beyond removal of or exemptions from fees, and instead transform the way tuberculosis diagnostic services are delivered.[11]

Russian Federation

The number of tuberculosis cases in the Russian Federation increased significantly during the 1990s; the number peaked in 2000, and has declined since. However, that decline is largely due to an effort to decrease tuberculosis cases in the prison population. Tuberculosis cases among the general public, particularly children, are still on the rise. DOTS is not widely used in this region, although tuberculosis case rates are down in the areas where it has been implemented.[12]

However, the government still has a strong commitment to controlling tuberculosis infection and has appointed a national body to address the issue of concurrent tuberculosis and HIV infection. Governmental agencies are also paying attention to the growing MDR-TB epidemic in the Russian Federation. Of particular concern is the growth of the Beijing strain of tuberculosis, which is not only drug-resistant, but is believed to be more virulent, more easily transmitted, and less susceptible to the Bacille Calmette-Guérin vaccine.[13]

Reduction of tuberculosis incidence, disability, and mortality is currently one of the priorities of state policy in the Russian Federation. A program called Prevention and Control of Social Diseases (2002–2006), with a subprogram called Urgent Measures of TB Control in Russia, was approved in 2001 and aims to stabilize the epidemiological situation of social diseases through improvement of current organizations and newly established services. The plan covers strengthening the capacities of health facilities, research institutes, and other organizations that carry out prevention, timely detection, diagnosis, and treatment.

Mexico

The National TB Control Program (NTCP) in Mexico began implementing the DOTS program in selected demonstration areas in Mexico in 1996, and by 2004 the DOTS population coverage was estimated to be 92%. However, in 2004 Mexico still had nearly 34,000 tuberculosis cases, with an estimated incidence rate of 32 cases per 100,000 people.[14] Health care workers in Mexico are particularly at risk: A four-year study found that the rate for health care workers in general was much higher than that for the general public—nearly 440 cases per 100,000 people. For physicians, the rate was 860 per 100,000, and for physicians in training it was more than 1,800 per 100,000.[15]

Mexico's tuberculosis rate is of particular concern to the United States because of our shared border and because of the high rate of immigration from Mexico. In fact, since 2001 about one quarter of the tuberculosis cases among non–U.S.-born people in the United States have been people from Mexico.[16] (Chapter 1 has more information about tuberculosis rates among immigrants.)

In 2000 the United States Agency for International Development (USAID) and the Mexican Secretariat of Health signed a $16 million bilateral grant agreement to strengthen efforts to control tuberculosis in Mexico; between 2000 and 2005, additional U.S. funds contributed to this program averaged $1.3 million per year. USAID and NTCP are also working together to target 13 Mexican states, including those along the U.S.-Mexico border and those with the highest tuberculosis rates and highest concentrations of migrants.[14] Since 2000, Mexico has met or exceeded the WHO's targets for treatment success and case detection.

This investment in tuberculosis control may bring economic benefits: One economic analysis showed that an investment of $35 million in tuberculosis control in Mexico by the United States would result in net discounted savings of $108 million over a 20-year period, through decreased costs associated with tuberculosis among Mexican immigrants to the United States.[17]

India

India carries the highest tuberculosis burden in the world: In 2005 the country had more than 1 million new and relapse cases, with an incidence rate of 168 per 100,000. About one third of all the world's tuberculosis cases are in India.

In addition, health care workers have a high risk of exposure. One study found that 50% of health care workers tested positive for LTBI by one of two tests, and 31% were positive on both tests.[18] This is of concern to the U.S. health system, as many Indian health care workers come to the United States to practice medicine.

To date, the United States has not provided any major funding for India's tuberculosis control efforts, although USAID has helped in the country's DOTS implementation. In addition, USAID has had significant involvement in India's HIV prevention and education program.

India's Revised National TB Control Program was introduced on a pilot scale in 1993 and was formally launched by the government in 1997. By mid-1998 the program had been expanded to serve about 20 million people. From that time until 2003, there was rapid growth in the DOTS program, so that by 2003 the areas covered by the DOTS strategy included 778 million people—approximately 67% of the population.[19]

Socially Excluded Groups in Europe

Ethnic groups that are excluded (or that intentionally exclude themselves) from general society tend to be at great risk for tuberculosis. The reasons for this include poverty as well as economic, cultural, geographical, and educational barriers to necessary health care services. Such is the case with the Roma.

The 12 million to 15 million Roma living in Eastern and Western Europe are sometimes referred to as *Gypsies,* although that term is considered pejorative (and may be partly to blame for some of the bigotry often experienced by this community). The Roma have historically suffered a great deal of discrimination: Various Romani groups have suffered persecution and ethnic cleansing since the fifteenth century; in the nineteenth century, many countries (including the United States) enacted laws forbidding Roma from immigrating; today, in some countries, Romani children are still segregated into separate, often inadequate, schools.

For these reasons, the Roma tend to live in isolated communities, far from primary health centers, and often distrust establishments and authority figures. These issues all put the Roma at higher risk for tuberculosis. Ministries of health in Eastern Europe do not collect data broken down by ethnic group, but a great deal of anecdotal evidence suggests that this group has tuberculosis rates that are two to seven times higher than the general population.[20] Therefore, governments and health agencies need to make a special effort to reach out to the Roma and other socially excluded groups to provide education and treatment, and to break down some of the economic and cultural barriers that prevent them from obtaining appropriate tuberculosis treatment.

Joint Commission International Standards

Joint Commission International (JCI) accreditation is a variety of initiatives designed to respond to a growing demand around the world for standards-based evaluation in health care. Its purpose is to offer the international community standards-based, objective processes for evaluating health care organizations. The goal of the program is to stimulate demonstration of continuous, sustained improvement in health care organizations by applying international consensus standards, International Patient Safety Goals, and indicator measurement support.[21]

The following requirements relate to care of patients, infection control measures, and environmental issues associated with tuberculosis.

Requirements Associated with Patient Assessment

1. Laboratory safety program
   - JCI requires that a laboratory safety program is in place, followed, and documented. The laboratory has an active safety program to the degree required by the risks and hazards encountered in the laboratory. The program addresses safety practices and prevention measures for laboratory staff, other staff, and patients when present.
   - The laboratory program is coordinated with the organization's safety management program.
   - The laboratory safety management program includes the following:
     - Written policies and procedures that support compliance with applicable standards and regulations
     - Written policies and procedures for the handling and disposal of infectious and hazardous materials
     - Availability of safety devices appropriate to the laboratory's practices and hazards encountered
     - The orientation of all laboratory staff to safety procedures and practices
     - In-service education for new procedures and newly acquired or recognized hazardous materials.

- The measurable elements for these requirements include the following:
  - A laboratory safety program is in place and is appropriate to the risks and hazards encountered.
  - The program is coordinated with the organization's safety management program.
  - Written policies and procedures address the handling and disposal of infectious and hazardous materials.
  - Appropriate safety devices are available.
  - Laboratory staff is oriented to safety procedures and practices.
  - Laboratory staff receives education for new procedures and newly acquired or recognized hazardous materials.
2. Radiation safety program
  - A radiation safety program should be in place, followed, and documented. The organization should have an active radiation safety program that includes all components of the organization's radiology and diagnostic imaging services, including radiation oncology and the cardiac catheterization laboratory. The radiation safety program reflects the risks and hazards encountered. The program addresses safety practices and prevention measures for radiology and diagnostic imaging staff, other staff, and patients.
  - The program should be coordinated with the organization's safety management program.
  - The radiation safety management program includes the following:
    - Written policies and procedures that support compliance with applicable standards, laws, and regulations
    - Written policies and procedures for handling and disposal of infectious and hazardous materials
    - Availability of safety protective devices appropriate to the practices and hazards encountered
    - The orientation of all radiology and diagnostic imaging staff to safety procedures and practices
    - In-service education for new procedures and newly acquired or recognized hazardous materials
  - The measurable elements for these requirements include the following:
    - A radiation safety program is in place and is appropriate to the risks and hazards encountered.
    - The program is coordinated with the organization's safety management program.

– Written policies and procedures address compliance with applicable standards, laws, and regulations.
– Written policies and procedures address handling and disposal of infectious and hazardous materials.
– Appropriate radiation safety devices are available.
– Radiology and diagnostic imaging staff are oriented to safety procedures and practices.
– Radiology and diagnostic imaging staff receive education for new procedures and hazardous materials.

Requirements Associated with Quality Improvement and Patient Safety

3. Data analysis
   - JCI requires that data are analyzed when undesirable trends and variation are evident from the data. When the organization detects or suspects undesirable change from what is expected, it initiates intense analysis to determine where best to focus improvement. In particular, intense analysis is initiated when levels, patterns, or trends vary significantly and undesirably from what was expected, from that of other organizations, or from recognized standards.
   - An analysis is conducted for the following:
     – All confirmed transfusion reactions, if applicable to the organization
     – All serious adverse drug events, if applicable and as defined by the organization
     – All significant medication errors, if applicable and as defined by the organization
     – All major discrepancies between preoperative and postoperative diagnoses
     – Adverse events or patterns of adverse events during moderate or deep sedation and anesthesia use
     – Other events such as infectious disease outbreaks
   - The measurable elements for these requirements include the following:
     – Intense analysis of data takes place when adverse levels, patterns, or trends occur.
     – All confirmed transfusion reactions, if applicable to the organization, are analyzed.
     – All serious adverse drug events, if applicable and as defined by the organization, are analyzed.
     – All significant medication errors, if applicable and as defined by the organization, are analyzed.
     – All major discrepancies between preoperative and postoperative diagnoses are analyzed.

- Adverse events or patterns of adverse events during moderate or deep sedation and anesthesia use are analyzed.
- Other events defined by the organization are analyzed.

Requirements Associated with Prevention and Control of Infections

4. Infection control program
   - JCI requires that an infection control program is based on current scientific knowledge, accepted practice guidelines, and applicable law and regulation. Information is essential to an infection control program. Current scientific information is required to understand and implement effective surveillance and control activities and can come from many national or international sources (for example, the WHO–published hand hygiene and other guidelines). Practice guidelines provide information on preventive practices and infections associated with clinical and support services. Applicable laws and regulations define elements of the basic program, the response to infectious disease outbreaks, and any reporting requirements.
   - The measurable elements for these requirements include the following:
     - The infection control program is based on current scientific knowledge.
     - The infection control program is based on accepted practice guidelines.
     - The infection control program is based on applicable laws and regulations.
5. Health care–associated infections
   - JCI requires that the organization designs and implements a comprehensive program to reduce the risks of health care–associated infections in patients and health care workers.
   - For an infection prevention and control program to be effective, it must be comprehensive, encompassing both patient care and employee health. The program is guided by a plan that identifies and addresses the infection issues that are epidemiologically important to the organization. In addition, the program and plan are appropriate to the organization's size and geographic location, services, and patients. The program includes systems to monitor infections and investigate outbreaks of infectious diseases. Policies and procedures guide the program. The periodic assessment of risk and setting of risk-reduction goals guide the program.
   - The measurable elements for these requirements include the following:
     - There is a comprehensive program and plan to reduce the risk of health care–associated infections in patients.
     - There is a comprehensive program and plan to reduce the risk of health care–associated infections in health care workers.

- The program includes systematic and proactive surveillance activities to determine usual (endemic) rates of infection.
- The program includes systems to investigate outbreaks of infectious diseases.
- The program is guided by appropriate policies and procedures.
- Risk-reduction goals and measurable objectives are established and regularly reviewed.
- The program is appropriate to the organization's size and geographic location, services, and patients.

6. Locations affected
   • JCI requires that all patient, staff, and visitor areas of the organization are included in the infection control program. Infections can enter the organization via patients, families, staff, volunteers, visitors, and other individuals such as trade representatives. Thus, all areas of the organization where these individuals are found must be included in the program of infection surveillance, prevention, and control.
   • The measurable elements for these requirements include the following:
     - All patient care areas of the organization are included in the infection control program.
     - All staff areas of the organization are included in the infection control program.
     - All visitor areas of the organization are included in the infection control program.

7. Focus of the program
   • JCI requires that the organization establishes the focus of the health care–associated infection prevention and reduction program. Each organization must identify those epidemiologically important infections, infection sites, and associated devices and procedures that will provide the focus of efforts to prevent and reduce the risk and incidence of health care–associated infections. Organizations consider, as appropriate, infections and processes that involve the following:
     - Respiratory tract—such as the procedures and equipment associated with intubation, mechanical ventilatory support, tracheostomy, and so on
     - Urinary tract—such as the invasive procedures and equipment associated with indwelling urinary catheters, urinary drainage systems, and their care, and so on
     - Intravascular invasive devices—such as the insertion and care of central venous catheters, peripheral venous lines, and so on
     - Surgical sites—such as their care and type of dressing and associated aseptic procedures

- Epidemiologically significant diseases and organisms—multidrug resistant organisms, highly virulent infections
- Emerging or reemerging infections with the community
- The measurable elements for these requirements include the following:
  - The organization has established the focus of the program to prevent or reduce the incidence of health care–associated infections.
  - Respiratory tract infections are included as appropriate to the organization.
  - Urinary tract infections are included as appropriate to the organization.
  - Intravascular invasive devices are included as appropriate to the organization.
  - Surgical wounds are included as appropriate to the organization.
  - Epidemiologically significant diseases and organisms are included as appropriate to the organization and its community.
  - Emerging or reemerging infections are included as appropriate to the organization and its community.

8. Risk identification and reduction
   - JCI requires that the organization identifies the procedures and processes associated with the risk of infection and implements strategies to reduce infection risk. Health care organizations assess and care for patients using many simple and complex processes, each associated with a level of infection risk to patients and staff. It is thus important for an organization to review and monitor those processes and, as appropriate, implement needed policies, procedures, education, and other activities to reduce the risk of infection.
   - The measurable elements for these requirements include the following:
     - The organization has identified those processes associated with infection risk.
     - The organization has implemented strategies to reduce infection risk in those processes.
     - The organization identifies which risks require policies and or procedures, staff education, practice changes, and other activities to support risk reduction.

9. Cleaning and disinfection
   - JCI requires the organization to reduce the risk of infections by ensuring adequate equipment cleaning and sterilization and the proper management of laundry and linen.
   - Infection risk is minimized with proper cleaning, disinfection, and sterilization processes, such as the cleaning and disinfection of endoscopes, sterilization of surgical supplies, and other invasive or noninvasive patient care equipment. Cleaning, disinfection, and sterilization can take place in a centralized sterilization area or in other areas of the organization, such as endoscope clinics, with

proper oversight. Also, the proper management of laundry and linen can result in reduced contamination of clean linen and reduced infection risk to staff from soiled laundry and linen.

- Infection risk increases with the reuse of single-use devices. When single-use devices are reused there is a hospital policy that guides such reuse. The policy is consistent with regulatory and professional standards. The policy includes identification of (1) devices and materials that can never be reused; (2) the maximum number of reuses for devices and materials that are reused; (3) the types of wear, cracking, and so forth, that indicate the device cannot be reused; (4) the cleaning process for devices that starts immediately after use and that follows a clear protocol; and (5) the process for the collection, analysis, and use of infection control data related to reused devices and materials.
- The measurable elements for these requirements include the following:
  - Equipment cleaning and sterilization methods in a central sterilization service are appropriate for the type of equipment.
  - Equipment cleaning, disinfection, and sterilization methods conducted outside of a central sterilization service are appropriate for the type of equipment.
  - When single-use devices and materials are reused, there is a policy that includes items (1) through (5) above, and the policy is implemented.
  - Laundry and linen management are appropriate to minimize risk to staff and patients.
  - There is a coordinated oversight process for all cleaning, disinfection, and sterilization throughout the organization.

10. Waste disposal
- JCI requires the organization to reduce the risk of infections through proper disposal of waste. Health care organizations produce considerable waste each day. Frequently that waste is or could be infectious. Thus, the proper disposal of waste contributes to the reduction of infection risk in the organization. This is true for the disposal of body fluids and materials contaminated with body fluids, the disposal of blood and blood components, and waste from the mortuary and postmortem areas, when present.
- The measurable elements associated with these requirements include the following:
  - Disposal of infectious waste and body fluids are managed to minimize transmission risk.
  - The handling and disposal of blood and blood components are managed to minimize transmission risk.

– Operation of the mortuary and postmortem area are managed to minimize transmission risk.

11. Barrier precautions and isolation procedures
- JCI requires the organization to provide barrier precautions and isolation procedures that protect patients, visitors, and staff from communicable diseases and protect immunosuppressed patients from acquiring infections to which they are uniquely prone. The organization develops policies and procedures that establish the isolation and barrier procedures for the hospital. These are based on the method of disease transmission and address individual patients who may be infectious or immunosuppressed, as well as the influx of large numbers of patients with contagious infections.
- The isolation procedures address staff and visitor protection, the patient environment, and the cleaning of the room during the stay and after the patient is discharged.
- The measurable elements associated with these requirements include the following:
  – Patients with known or suspected contagious diseases are isolated in accordance with organization policy and recommended guidelines.
  – Policies and procedures address the separation of patients with communicable diseases from patients and staff who are at greater risk due to immunosuppression or other reasons.
  – The organization has a strategy of dealing with an influx of patients with contagious diseases
  – Appropriate negative-pressure rooms are available and monitored routinely for infectious patients who require isolation.
  – Staff are educated in the management of infectious patients.

Requirements Associated with Governance, Leadership, and Direction

12. Community interaction
- JCI requires organization leaders plan with community leaders and leaders of other organizations to meet the community's health care needs. An organization's mission commonly reflects the needs of the population in its community. Similarly, referral and specialty care organizations derive their missions from the needs of patients within larger geographic or political areas.
- The needs of patients and communities usually change over time, and thus, health care organizations need to engage their communities in the strategic and operational planning of the organization. Organizations do this by seeking

opinions or input on an individual or group basis through advisory groups or task forces, for example.

- Thus, it is important for the leaders of a health care organization to meet with, and plan with, recognized community leaders and the leaders of other provider organizations in the community. The leaders plan for a healthier community and recognize that they have responsibility for and an impact on the community, even in the absence of such planning.
- The measurable elements associated with these requirements include the following:
  - The organization's leaders plan with recognized community leaders.
  - The organization's leaders plan with the leaders of other provider organizations in its community.
  - The organization's leaders seek the input of individual and group stakeholders in its community as part of its strategic and operational planning.
  - The organization participates in community education on health promotion and disease prevention.

Requirements Associated with the Care of Patients

13. Patient care
    - JCI requires that policies and procedures guide the following:
      - Care of emergency patients
      - The use of resuscitation services throughout the organization
      - The handling, use, and administration of blood and blood products
      - The care of patients on life support or who are comatose
      - The care of patients with a communicable disease and immune-suppressed patients
      - The care of patients on dialysis
      - Use of restraint and the care of patients in restraint
      - The care of elderly patients, disabled individuals, children, and populations at risk for abuse
      - The care of patients receiving chemotherapy or other high-risk medications
    - Policies and procedures must be tailored to the particular at-risk patient population or high-risk service to be appropriate and effective in reducing the related risk. It is particularly important that the policy or procedure identify the following:
      - How planning will occur, including the identification of differences between adult and pediatric populations, or other special considerations
      - The documentation required for the care team to work and communicate effectively

- Special consent considerations, if appropriate
- Patient monitoring requirements
- Special qualifications or skills of staff involved in the care process
- The availability and use of specialized equipment
- Clinical guidelines and clinical pathways are frequently helpful in developing the policies and procedures and may be incorporated into them.
- The measurable elements associated with these requirements include the following:
  - The care of patients with a communicable disease is guided by appropriate policies and procedures.
  - The care of immune-suppressed patients is guided by appropriate policies and procedures.
  - Immune-suppressed patients and patients with communicable diseases receive care according to the policies and procedures.

Requirements Associated with Staff Qualifications and Education

14. Staff safety and health program
    - JCI requires an organization to provide a staff health and safety program. The health and safety of an organization's staff are important to maintain staff satisfaction and productivity. Staff safety is also a part of the organization's quality and patient safety program. How an organization orients and trains staff, provides a safe workplace, maintains biomedical and other equipment, prevents or controls health care–associated infections, and many other factors determines the health and well-being of staff.
    - A staff health and safety program can be located within the organization or be integrated into external programs. Whatever the staffing and structure of the program, staff understand how to report, be treated for, and receive counseling and follow-up for injuries such as needlesticks, exposure to infectious diseases, identification of risks and hazardous conditions in the facility, and other health and safety matters. The program may also provide for initial employment health screening, periodic preventive immunizations and examinations, and treatment for common work-related conditions, such as back injuries, or more urgent injuries.
    - The design of the program includes staff input and draws upon the organization's clinical resources as well as those in the community.
    - The measurable elements associated with these requirements include the following:

- The organization's leaders and staff plan the health and safety program.
- The program is responsive to urgent and nonurgent staff needs through direct treatment and referral.
- Program data inform the organization's quality and safety program.
- There is a policy on the provision of staff vaccinations and immunizations.
- There is a policy on the evaluation, counseling, and follow-up of staff exposed to infectious diseases that is coordinated with the infection prevention and control program.

References

1. World Health Organization: *Global Plan to Stop TB 2006–2015.* http://www.who.int/tb/en/ (accessed Jul. 11, 2007).
2. Altman L.K.: Doctors warn of powerful and resistant tuberculosis strain. *New York Times,* Aug. 18, 2007. http://query.nytimes.com/gst/fullpage.html?res=9B0DE0D6143EF93BA2575BC0A9609C8B63 (accessed Oct. 4, 2007).
3. Raviglione M.C., Pio A.: Evolution of WHO policies for tuberculosis control. *Lancet* 359:775–780, 2002.
4. World Health Organization: *Pursue High-Quality DOTS Expansion and Enhancement.* http://www.who.int/tb/dots/en/ (accessed Jul. 12, 2007).
5. World Health Organization: *An Expanded DOTS Framework for Effective Tuberculosis Control.* http://www.who.int/tb/publications/expanded_dots_framework/en/ (accessed Jul. 12, 2007).
6. Migliori G.B., et al.: Extensively drug-resistant tuberculosis, Italy and Germany. *Emerg Infect Dis* 13, May 2007. http://www.cdc.gov/EID/content/13/5/780.htm (accessed Jul. 12, 2007).
7. Centers for Disease Control and Prevention: *CDC Health Information for International Travel, 2008.* http://wwwn.cdc.gov/travel/contentYellowBook.aspx (accessed Jul. 12, 2007).
8. Pan American Health Organization: *Regional Plan for Tuberculosis Control, 2006–2015.* http://www.paho.org/English/AD/DPC/CD/tb-reg-plan-2006-15.pdf (accessed Jul. 12, 2007).
9. World Lung Foundation: *China.* http://www.worldlungfoundation.org/map_china.html (accessed Jul. 1, 2007).
10. Kapp C.: XDR tuberculosis spreads across South Africa. *Lancet.* 369:729, 2007.
11. Kemp J.R., et al.: Can Malawi's poor afford free tuberculosis services? Patient and household costs associated with a tuberculosis diagnosis in Lilongwe. *Bull World Health Organ* 85:580–585, Aug. 2007.
12. World Lung Foundation: *Russian Federation.* http://www.worldlungfoundation.org/map_Russian.html (accessed Jul. 1, 2007).
13. Drobniewski F., et al.: Drug-resistant tuberculosis, clinical virulence, and the dominance of the Beijing strain family in Russia. *JAMA* 293:2726–2731, Jun. 8, 2005.

14. United States Agency for International Development: *Mexico: Tuberculosis Profile.* Sep. 2006. http://www.usaid.gov/our_work/global_health/id/tuberculosis/countries/lac/mexico_profile.html (accessed Jul. 12, 2007).

15. Laniado-Laborín R., Cabrales-Vargas N.: Tuberculosis in healthcare workers at a general hospital in Mexico. *Infect Control Hosp Epidemiol* 27:449–452, May 2006.

16. Centers for Disease Control and Prevention (CDC): *Reported Tuberculosis in the United States, 2005.* Atlanta: U.S. Department of Health and Human Services, CDC, 2006.

17. Schwartzman K., et al.: Domestic returns from investment in the control of tuberculosis in other countries. *N Engl J Med* 353:32–44, 2005.

18. Pai M.: *Mycobacterium tuberculosis* infection in health care workers in rural India. *JAMA* 293:2746–2755, Jun 8, 2005.

19. World Lung Foundation: *India.* http://www.worldlungfoundation.org/map_india.html (accessed Jul. 1, 2007).

20. Schaaf M.: *Confronting a Hidden Disease: TB in Roma Communities.* New York: Open Society Institute, 2007.

21. Joint Commission Resources: *Joint Commission International Accreditation Standards for Hospitals,* 3rd ed.. Oakbrook Terrace, IL: The Joint Commission, 2008.

Glossary

Adapted from Centers for Disease Control and Prevention: Guidelines for preventing the transmission of *Mycobacterium tuberculosis* in health-care settings, 2005. *MMWR Recomm Rep* 54:1–147, Dec. 30, 2005.

acid-fast bacilli (AFB) examination

A laboratory test that involves microscopic examination of a stained smear of a patient specimen (usually sputum) to determine if mycobacteria are present. A presumptive diagnosis of pulmonary tuberculosis can be made with a positive AFB sputum smear result; however, approximately 50% of patients with tuberculosis disease of the lungs have negative AFB sputum smear results. The diagnosis of tuberculosis disease is usually not confirmed until *Mycobacterium tuberculosis* is identified in culture or by a positive nucleic acid amplification (NAA) test result.

aerosol

Dispersions of particles in a gaseous medium (for example, air). Droplet nuclei are an example of particles that are expelled by a person with an infectious disease (for example, by coughing, sneezing, or singing). For *M. tuberculosis,* the droplet nuclei are approximately 1–5 μm. Because of their small size, the droplet nuclei can remain suspended in the air for substantial periods and can transmit *M. tuberculosis* to other persons.

AII room

A room designed to maintain AII. Formerly called negative pressure isolation room, an AII room is a single-occupancy patient-care room used to isolate persons with suspected or confirmed infectious tuberculosis disease. Environmental factors are controlled in AII rooms to minimize the transmission of infectious agents that are usually spread from person to person by droplet nuclei associated with coughing or aerosolization of contaminated fluids. AII rooms should provide negative pressure in the room (so that air flows under the door gap into the room), an airflow rate of 6–12 ACH, and direct exhaust of air from the room to the outside of the building or recirculation of air through a high-efficiency particulate air (HEPA) filter.

airborne infection isolation (AII)

The isolation of patients infected with organisms that spread through airborne droplet nuclei 1–5 μm in diameter. This isolation area receives substantial ACH (> 12 ACH for new construction since 2001 and > 6 ACH for construction before 2001) and is under negative pressure (for example, the direction of the airflow is from the outside adjacent space [for example, the corridor] into the room). The air in an AII room is preferably exhausted to the outside but can be recirculated if the return air is filtered through a HEPA filter.

air change

Ratio of the airflow in volume units per hour to the volume of the space under consideration in identical volume units, usually expressed in air changes per hour (ACH).

air changes per hour (ACH)

Air change rate expressed as the number of air exchange units per hour.

aminotransaminases

Also called transaminases. Used to assess for hepatotoxicity in persons taking antituberculosis medications; they include aspartate amino transferase (AST), serum glutamic oxalacetic transaminase (formerly SGOT), and amino alanine transferase (formerly ALT).

anergy

A condition in which a person has a diminished ability to exhibit delayed T-cell hypersensitivity to antigens because of a condition or situation resulting in altered immune function.

Bacille Calmette-Guérin

A vaccine for tuberculosis, named after the French scientists Calmette and Guérin, used in most countries where tuberculosis disease is endemic. The vaccine is effective in preventing disseminated and meningeal tuberculosis disease in infants and young children. It may have approximately 50% efficacy for preventing pulmonary tuberculosis disease in adults.

baseline tuberculosis screening

The screening of health care workers for latent tuberculosis infection (LTBI) and tuberculosis disease at the beginning of employment. Tuberculosis screening includes a symptom screen for all health care workers, and tuberculin skin tests (TSTs) or blood assay for *Mycobacterium tuberculosis* (BAMT) for those with previous negative test results for *M. tuberculosis* infection.

baseline TST or baseline BAMT

The TST or BAMT administered at the beginning of employment to newly hired health care workers. If the TST method is used, for health care workers who have not had a documented negative test result for *M. tuberculosis* during the preceding 12 months, the baseline TST result should be obtained by using the two-step method. BAMT baseline testing does not require the two-step method.

blood assay for *Mycobacterium tuberculosis* (BAMT)

A general term referring to recently developed in vitro diagnostic tests that assess for the presence of infection with *M. tuberculosis*. This term includes, but is not limited to, interferon-γ (interferon-gamma) release assays.

BAMT converter

A change from a negative to a positive BAMT result over a two-year period.

bronchoscopy

A procedure for examining the lower respiratory tract in which the end of the endoscopic instrument is inserted through the mouth or nose (or tracheostomy) and into the respiratory tree. Bronchoscopy can be used to obtain diagnostic specimens. Bronchoscopy also creates a high risk for *M. tuberculosis* transmission to health care workers if it is performed on an untreated patient who has tuberculosis disease (even if the patient has negative AFB smear results) because it is a cough-inducing procedure.

cluster

A group of patients with LTBI or tuberculosis disease that are linked by epidemiologic, location, or genotyping data. Two or more TST conversions within a short period can be a cluster of tuberculosis disease and might suggest transmission within the setting. A genotyping cluster is two or more cases with isolates that have an identical genotyping pattern.

contact
Refers to someone who was exposed to *M. tuberculosis* infection by sharing air space with an infectious tuberculosis patient.

contact investigation
Procedures that occur when a case of infectious tuberculosis is identified, including finding persons (contacts) exposed to the case, testing and evaluation of contacts to identify LTBI or tuberculosis disease, and treatment of these persons, as indicated.

conversion
See TST conversion.

conversion rate
The percentage of a population with a converted test result (TST or BAMT) for *M. tuberculosis* within a specified period. This is calculated by dividing the number of conversions among eligible health care workers in the setting in a specified period (numerator) by the number of health care workers who received tests in the setting over the same period (denominator), multiplied by 100.

cough etiquette
See respiratory hygiene and cough etiquette.

culture
Growth of microorganisms in the laboratory performed for detection and identification in sputum or other body fluids and tissues. This test usually takes two to four weeks for mycobacteria to grow (two to four days for most other bacteria).

directly observed therapy (DOT)
Adherence-enhancing strategy in which a health care worker or other trained person watches as a patient swallows each dose of medication. DOT is the standard care for all patients with tuberculosis disease and is a preferred option for patients treated for LTBI.

directly observed therapy, short course (DOTS)
A comprehensive adherence-enhancing strategy that includes DOT as well as additional methods to promote treatment adherence, such as providing support and care that emphasizes the needs of the individual patients and their families and finding locally appropriate ways to motivate patients to participate in and complete tuberculosis treatment.

droplet nuclei
Microscopic particles produced when a person coughs, sneezes, shouts, or sings. These particles can remain suspended in the air for prolonged periods and can be carried on normal air currents in a room and beyond to adjacent spaces or areas receiving exhaust air.

drug susceptibility test
A laboratory determination to assess whether an *M. tuberculosis* complex isolate is susceptible or resistant to antituberculosis drugs that are added to mycobacterial growth medium or are detected genetically. The results predict whether a specific drug is likely to be effective in treating tuberculosis disease caused by that isolate.

exposure
A situation in which persons (for example, health care workers, visitors, inmates) have been exposed to a person with suspected or confirmed infectious tuberculosis disease (or to air containing *M. tuberculosis*), without the benefit of effective infection control measures.

extrapulmonary tuberculosis
Tuberculosis disease in any part of the body other than the lungs (for example, kidney, spine, lymph nodes). The presence of extrapulmonary disease does not exclude pulmonary tuberculosis disease.

fit test
The use of a protocol to qualitatively or quantitatively evaluate the fit of a respirator on a person. A qualitative fit test is a pass/fail fit test to assess the adequacy of respirator fit that relies on the response of the person to the test agent; a quantitative fit test is an assessment of the adequacy of respirator fit by numerically measuring the amount of leakage into the respirator.

infection control program
A program designed to control transmission of *M. tuberculosis* through early detection, isolation, and treatment of persons with infectious tuberculosis. A hierarchy of control measures are used, including (1) administrative controls to reduce the risk of exposure to persons with infectious tuberculosis disease and increase screening for health care workers for LTBI and tuberculosis disease, (2) environmental controls to prevent the spread and reduce the concentration of infectious droplet nuclei in the

air, and (3) respiratory protection in areas where the risk for exposure to *M. tuberculosis* is high (for example, AII rooms). A tuberculosis infection control plan should include surveillance of health care workers who have unprotected high-risk exposure to tuberculosis patients or their environment of care.

health care–associated
Acquired in a health care facility; broader term used instead of *nosocomial.*

health care setting
A place where health care is delivered.

health care workers
All paid and unpaid persons working in health care settings.

hemoptysis
The expectoration or coughing up of blood or blood-tinged sputum; one of the symptoms of pulmonary tuberculosis disease. Hemoptysis can also be observed in other pulmonary conditions (for example, lung cancer).

high-efficiency particulate air (HEPA) filter
A filter that is certified to remove > 99.97% of particles 0.3 μm in size, including *M. tuberculosis*–containing droplet nuclei; the filter can be either portable or stationary. Use of HEPA filters in building ventilation systems requires expertise in installation and maintenance.

human immunodeficiency virus (HIV) infection
Infection with the virus that causes acquired immunodeficiency syndrome (AIDS). A person with both LTBI and HIV infection is at high risk for developing tuberculosis disease.

immunocompromised and immunosuppressed
Describes conditions in which at least part of the immune system is functioning at less than normal capacity. According to certain style experts, *immunocompromised* is the broader term, and *immunosuppressed* is restricted to conditions with iatrogenic causes, including treatments for another condition.

incidence

The number of new events or cases of disease that develop during a specified period.

index case

The first person with tuberculosis disease identified in a particular setting. This person might be an indicator of a potential public health problem and is not necessarily the source case. *See also* source case or patient.

induration

The firmness in the skin test reaction; produced by immune cell infiltration in response to the tuberculin antigen that was introduced into the skin. Induration is measured transversely by palpation, and the result is recorded in millimeters. The measurement is compared with guidelines to determine whether the test result is classified as positive or negative.

infectious droplet nuclei

Droplet nuclei produced by an infectious tuberculosis patient that can carry tubercle bacteria and can be inhaled by others. Although usually produced from patients with pulmonary tuberculosis through coughing, aerosol-generating procedures can also generate infectious droplet nuclei.

infectious period

The period during which a person with tuberculosis disease might have transmitted *M. tuberculosis* organisms to others. For patients with positive AFB sputum smear results, the infectious period begins three months before the collection date of the first positive smear result or the symptom onset date (whichever is earlier) and ends when the patient is placed into AII or the date of collection for the first of consistently negative smear results. For patients with negative AFB sputum smear results, the infectious period extends from one month before the symptom onset date and ends when the patient is placed into AII.

isoniazid

A highly active antituberculosis chemotherapeutic agent that is a cornerstone of treatment for tuberculosis disease and the cornerstone of treatment for LTBI.

laryngeal tuberculosis
A form of tuberculosis disease that involves the larynx and that can be highly infectious.

latent tuberculosis infection (LTBI)
Infection with *M. tuberculosis* without symptoms or signs of disease having manifested.

Mantoux method
A skin test performed by intradermally injecting 0.1 mL of purified protein derivative (PPD) tuberculin solution into the volar or dorsal surface of the forearm. This is the recommended method for TST.

mask
A device worn over the nose and mouth of a person with suspected or confirmed infectious tuberculosis disease to prevent infectious particles from being released into room air.

miliary tuberculosis
A serious form of tuberculosis disease sometimes referred to as disseminated tuberculosis. A dangerous and difficult form to diagnose of rapidly progressing tuberculosis disease that extends throughout the body. Uniformly fatal if untreated; in certain instances, it is diagnosed too late to save a life. Certain patients with this condition have normal findings or ordinary infiltrates on the chest radiograph.

multidrug-resistant tuberculosis
Tuberculosis disease caused by *M. tuberculosis* organisms that are resistant to at least isoniazid and rifampin.

Mycobacterium tuberculosis
The namesake member organism of *M. tuberculosis* complex and the most common causative infectious agent of tuberculosis disease in humans. In certain instances, the species name refers to the entire *M. tuberculosis* complex, which includes *M. bovis, M. african, M. microti, M. canetii, M. caprae,* and *M. pinnipedii.*

N95 respirator mask
An air-purifying, filtering-facepiece respirator that is > 95% efficient at removing 0.3 μm particles and that is not resistant to oil. *See* also respirator.

negative pressure
The difference in air pressure between two areas. A room that is under negative pressure has a lower pressure than adjacent areas, which keeps air from flowing out of the room and into adjacent rooms or areas. Also used to describe a nonpowered respirator. *See also* AII room and airborne infection isolation.

nosocomial
Acquired in a hospital. The broader term *health care–associated* is used in the Centers for Disease Control and Prevention (CDC) guidelines.

nucleic acid amplification (NAA)
Laboratory method used to target and amplify a single DNA or RNA sequence, usually for detecting and identifying a microorganism. The NAA tests for *M. tuberculosis* complex are sensitive and specific and can accelerate the confirmation of pulmonary tuberculosis disease.

potential ongoing transmission
A risk classification for tuberculosis screening, including testing for *M. tuberculosis* infection when evidence of ongoing transmission of *M. tuberculosis* is apparent in the setting. Testing might need to be performed every 8–10 weeks until lapses in infection controls have been corrected and until no further evidence of ongoing transmission is apparent. Use *potential ongoing transmission* as a temporary risk classification only. After corrective steps are taken, reclassify the setting as medium risk. Maintaining the classification of *medium risk* for at least one year is recommended.

powered air-purifying respirator (PAPR)
A respirator equipped with a tight-fitting facepiece (rubber facepiece) or loose-fitting facepiece (hood or helmet), breathing tube, air-purifying filter, cartridge or canister, and fan. Air is drawn through the air-purifying element and pushed through the breathing tube and into the facepiece, hood, or helmet by the fan. Loose-fitting PAPRs (for example, hoods or helmets) might be useful for persons with facial hair because they do not require a tight seal with the face.

pulmonary tuberculosis
Tuberculosis disease that occurs in the lung parenchyma, usually producing a cough that lasts more than three weeks.

purified protein derivative (PPD)
A material used in diagnostic tests for detecting infection with *M. tuberculosis.* In the United States, PPD tuberculin solution is approved for administration as an intradermal injection (5 TU per 0.1 mL), a diagnostic aid for LTBI [*see* tuberculin skin test (TST)].

recirculation
Ventilation in which all or the majority of the air exhausted from an area is returned to the same area or other areas of the setting.

respirator
A CDC/National Institute for Occupational Safety and Health–approved device worn to prevent inhalation of airborne contaminants.

respiratory hygiene and cough etiquette
Procedures by which patients with suspected or confirmed infectious tuberculosis disease can minimize the spread of infectious droplet nuclei by decreasing the number of infectious particles that are released into the environment. Patients with a cough should be instructed to turn their heads away from persons and to cover their mouth and nose with their hands or preferably with a cloth or tissue when coughing or sneezing.

rifampin
A highly active antituberculosis chemotherapeutic agent that is a cornerstone of treatment for tuberculosis disease.

risk assessment
An initial and ongoing evaluation of the risk for transmission of *M. tuberculosis* in a particular health care setting. To perform a risk assessment, the following factors should be considered: the community rate of tuberculosis; the number of tuberculosis patients encountered in the setting; and the speed with which patients with tuberculosis disease are suspected, isolated, and evaluated. The tuberculosis risk assessment determines the types of administrative and environmental controls and respiratory protection needed for a setting.

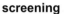

screening
Measures used to identify persons who have tuberculosis disease or LTBI; also, an administrative control measure in which evaluation for LTBI and tuberculosis disease are performed through initial and serial screening of health care workers, as indicated. Evaluation might comprise TST, BAMT, chest radiograph, and symptom screening.

screening program
A plan that health care settings should implement to provide information that is critical in caring for health care workers and that facilitates detection of *M. tuberculosis* transmission. The tuberculosis screening program comprises four major components: (1) baseline testing for *M. tuberculosis* infection, (2) serial testing for *M. tuberculosis* infection, (3) serial screening for signs or symptoms of tuberculosis disease, and (4) tuberculosis training and education.

source case or patient
The person or the case that was the original source of infection for secondary cases or contacts. The source case can be, but is not necessarily, the index case.

sputum
Mucus containing secretions coughed up from inside the lungs. Tests of sputum (for example, smear, culture) can confirm pulmonary tuberculosis disease. Sputum is different from saliva or nasal secretions, which are unsatisfactory specimens for detecting tuberculosis disease. However, specimens suspected to be inadequate should still be processed because positive culture results can still be obtained and might be the only bacteriologic indication of disease.

sputum induction
A method used to obtain sputum from a patient who is unable to cough up a specimen spontaneously. The patient inhales a saline mist, which stimulates coughing from deep inside the lungs.

transmission
Any mode or mechanism by which an infectious agent is spread from a source through the environment or to a person (or other living organism). In the context of health care–associated tuberculosis infection control, transmission is the airborne conveyance of aerosolized *M. tuberculosis* contained in droplet nuclei from a person with tuberculosis disease, usually from the respiratory tract, to another person, resulting in infection.

treatment

Treatment that prevents the progression of infection into disease.

TST conversion

A change in the result of a test for *M. tuberculosis* infection wherein the condition is interpreted as having progressed from uninfected to infected. An increase of > 10 mm in induration during a maximum of two years is defined as a TST conversion for the purposes of a contact investigation. TST conversion is presumptive evidence of new *M. tuberculosis* infection and poses an increased risk for progression to tuberculosis disease. *See also* conversion.

tubercle bacilli

M. tuberculosis organisms.

tuberculin

A precipitate made from a sterile filtrate of *M. tuberculosis* culture medium.

tuberculin skin test (TST)

A diagnostic aid for finding *M. tuberculosis* infection. A small dose of tuberculin is injected just beneath the surface of the skin (in the United States by the Mantoux method), and the area is examined for induration by palpation 48–72 hours after the injection. The indurated margins should be read transverse (perpendicular) to the long axis of the forearm. *See also* Mantoux method and purified protein derivative (PPD).

tuberculosis disease

Condition caused by infection with a member of the *M. tuberculosis* complex that has progressed to causing clinical (manifesting symptoms or signs) or subclinical (early stage of disease in which signs or symptoms are not present, but other indications of disease activity are present) illness. The bacteria can attack any part of the body, but disease is most commonly found in the lungs (pulmonary tuberculosis). Pulmonary tuberculosis disease can be infectious, whereas extrapulmonary disease (occurring at a body site outside the lungs) is not infectious, except in rare circumstances. When the only clinical finding is specific chest radiographic abnormalities, the condition is termed *inactive tuberculosis* and can be differentiated from active tuberculosis disease, which is accompanied by symptoms or other indications of disease activity (for example, the ability to culture reproducing tuberculosis organisms from respiratory secretions or specific chest radiographic findings).

two-step TST

Procedure used for the baseline skin testing of persons who will receive serial TSTs (for example, health care workers, residents or staff of correctional facilities or long term care facilities) to reduce the likelihood of mistaking a boosted reaction for a new infection. If an initial TST result is classified as negative, the second step of a two-step TST should be administered one to three weeks after the first TST result was read. If the second TST result is positive, it probably represents a boosted reaction, indicating infection most likely occurred in the past and not recently. If the second TST result is also negative, the person is classified as not infected. Two-step skin testing has no place in contact investigations or in other circumstances in which ongoing transmission of *M. tuberculosis* is suspected.

ultraviolet germicidal irradiation (UVGI)

Use of ultraviolet irradiation to kill or inactivate microorganisms.

Index